Effectively Managing Patient Education

GOING BEYOND
JOINT COMMISSION REQUIREMENTS

SUSAN KANACK

Effectively Managing Patient Education: Going Beyond Joint Commission Requirements
is published by HCPro, Inc.

Copyright © 2009 HCPro, Inc.

ISBN: 978-1-60146-319-7

Susan Kanack, BSN, RN, Author
Heather Comak, Managing Editor
Brian Driscoll, Executive Editor
Bob Croce, Group Publisher
Brenda Rossi, Cover Designer
Jackie Diehl Singer, Graphic Artist

Audrey Doyle, Copyeditor
Claire Cloutier, Proofreader
Darren Kelly, Books Production Supervisor
Susan Darbyshire, Art Director
Jean St. Pierre, Director of Operations

Advice given is general. Readers should consult professional counsel for specific legal, ethical, or clinical questions. Arrangements can be made for quantity discounts. For more information, contact:

HCPro, Inc.
P.O. Box 1168
Marblehead, MA 01945
Telephone: 800/650-6787 or 781/639-1872
Fax: 781/639-2982
E-mail: *customerservice@hcpro.com*

Visit HCPro at its World Wide Web sites:
www.hcpro.com and *www.hcmarketplace.com*

Contents

Figure List

© 2009 HCPro, Inc.
Effectively Managing Patient Education

About the Author

Susan Kanack, BSN, RN

Susan Kanack, BSN, RN, is the system coordinator for patient education at ProHealth Care. Based in Waukesha, WI, ProHealth Care is a healthcare organization comprising two inpatient hospital facilities, 27 primary care clinics, home health services, long-term care, and a health and fitness center. She manages patient education at a strategic and operational level for the organization.

Prior to ProHealth Care, Kanack worked as a labor and delivery nurse in several urban hospitals within the Milwaukee metropolitan area, as well as developed and coordinated educational activities at an organizational level for staff members and physicians. She obtained her bachelor of science degree in nursing from Carroll-Columbia College of Nursing in Waukesha in 1998, and has been an RN for more than 10 years.

Kanack is a certified Change Agent and has been instrumental in spearheading culture change within her organization related to patient education practices. She sits on the board of directors for the Literacy Council of Greater Waukesha and is a member of the Southeast Regional Health Literacy Committee for the state of Wisconsin. She is also a member of the Health Care Education Association.

She has contributed to several articles and publications on patient education and has spoken at several conferences.

Dedication

To my dad, Kenneth R. Strozyk, who always made me feel like I could do anything that I put my mind to.

To the loves of my life, Ian Parker Kanack and Sofia Grace Kanack: *Dream Big*. The world is yours.

Acknowledgments

I could not have written this book without the knowledge, assistance, and friendship of the following people who have mentored me and provided guidance, wisdom, talent, and encouragement:

Janet Schulz

Ann Woodward

Rebecca Hay

Christopher Scherer

Monica Erdmann

Tina T. Smith

Jennifer Anderson

Heather Comak

Linda Oddan

Vicki Kuenzi

Patrick Mullen

And finally, my accomplishments mean absolutely nothing to me without the love and support of my best friend and husband, Aaron Kanack; my mom, Diane Strozyk; and my sister, Donna Wagner. Love you all.

Introduction

It's time for patient education to enter the spotlight. It's been lying dormant for too long; passed over in favor of other competing priorities; wrapped up in other initiatives; or simply laid at the feet of a patient education manager to analyze and execute on his or her own. Patient education, a concept that staff members often view as more of a task than a process, is one of the few responsibilities that is shared across healthcare disciplines and involves virtually all healthcare professions. It's a process that often is minimized to a standardized checklist and a "one-size-fits-all" paradigm, an approach that is a tremendous disservice to patients and their families. Now is the time to take a step back, redefine your work, redefine patient education, and redefine what it means to provide this critical aspect of patient care in healthcare today.

Patient education means more than just meeting Joint Commission requirements; it means patient safety, patient and staff member satisfaction, marketability, and community image. It's linked directly to and embodied in patient- and family-centered care, health literacy, culturally competent care, and linguistic services. In fact, in its broadest definition, patient education can mean just about any healthcare communication from provider to patient. Unlike a procedure, which may occur only once a month in the hospital setting, patient education and communication with patients and their families occurs on a daily basis. As a result, this critical element in healthcare needs to be examined, thoroughly, and within the larger context of the healthcare industry and your hospital. It's time to engage your organization. Let the journey begin.

Analyzing Patient Education

Patients, their families, and regulatory agencies such as The Joint Commission and the Institute for Healthcare Improvement are demanding more from healthcare providers. Like healthcare itself, patients have evolved; thus, our care for them, including the education we provide to them, must evolve as well.

To better understand this evolution, it's important to look at the history of healthcare.

Understanding healthcare trends

The existence of hospitals in the United States date back to the eighteenth century. A hospital's purpose in the 1700s was to shelter the dying, orphans, and seafarers, and to prevent the spread of communicable diseases. As the U.S. population grew, mental illness added to the burdens of the country's inhabitants. Individuals whose behavior offended or frightened the general public were reported to the town board, which then ordered the individual's family to build a "strong house" or cell in which to house the individual on their property. If family or friends were unavailable, the person was auctioned to the lowest bidder, who would then have to care for that person, many times in exchange for physical labor.[1]

With the spread of contagious diseases, townships began to isolate infectious individuals. As that practice grew, "sick houses" (or isolation hospitals, as they were named) suddenly provided an ideal method for dealing with the homeless, petty criminals, and, eventually, the mentally ill. Hospitals during this period were never intended for the general population to use. Medical care was, for the most part, provided in the home.[1]

It's interesting to note that many hospitals today have a history that chronicles the evolution of healthcare quite well. The Poor House of New York City, established in 1736, was originally created to house the "poor, aged, insane, and disreputable." Today, it is known as the prestigious Bellevue Hospital. The Public Hospital of Baltimore, established in 1789, was home to low-income earners and people with mental illness, disabilities, and other physical ailments. One hundred years later, in 1889, it became the renowned Johns Hopkins Hospital.[1]

Understanding patient trends

As stated earlier, hospitals and healthcare delivery are not the only things that have evolved; patients have as well. The "sick role," described by Talcott Parsons in 1951, refers to the paternalistic, authoritarian relationship between a patient and his or her healthcare provider.[1] This theory, described by Frederick Wolinksy as "an integral part of the sociocultural definition of health and illness,"[1] was the model for healthcare interactions in which a patient complacently listened to the advice of his or her doctor, following orders and taking whatever medicines or treatments were prescribed. Most healthcare practitioners have been taught, and subsequently practice, in this manner; they hold the answers, and the patient's duty is to follow their recommendations to get better.

                        Effectively Managing Patient Education

Today, encouraging patients to engage in their healthcare and promoting more of a "partnership" between providers and patients is the mainstream; patients tend to "prefer participatory medical decision-making in their treatment, particularly educated patients."[2] Additionally, many patients have identified that they prefer clear communication, an ongoing (as opposed to episodic) doctor–patient relationship, and the feeling of empowerment.[3] Such trends, as well as the larger movement toward patient- and family-centered care, are bringing patient education into the spotlight.

About This Book

This book, targeted to individuals in centralized patient education roles, is designed to provide the insight, experience, and tools necessary to take patient education to the next level. Incorporating regulatory agency standards, patient safety organization recommendations, and tried and true leadership theories, this book will equip patient education managers with the tools and skills they need to evolve their patient education programs to a much larger initiative beyond simply providing patient education materials.

In healthcare today, many priorities are competing to gain the attention of senior leaders and staff members. The patient education manager needs to be politically savvy to navigate this situation and to advocate for patient education. In this book, I provide tips on how to talk to leaders, implement and navigate through the change process, obtain organizational support and buy-in, and understand what The Joint Commission and other organizations require; tips which I've gathered from my experience instituting patient education in my organization.

Like many things, evolving a program from point A to point B can be a challenge; often, such changes require many years, and sometimes leadership turnover, to come to fruition. But by being equipped with the right tools, you can jump-start those changes and pave the way for much larger accomplishments in the future. Change does not happen overnight; groundwork must be laid, and the patient education manager must lay that groundwork.

I hope you will learn from my experience in patient education and bring your organization to the next level of this important and necessary aspect of patient care.

References

1. Sultz, H., and Young, K. *Health Care USA: Understanding Its Organization and Delivery.* Sudbury, MA: Jones & Bartlett Publishers, Inc., 2008, p. 72–74.

2. Ryan, J., and Sysko, J. "The contingency of patient preferences for involvement in health decision making." *Health Care Management Review* 32 (2007): p. 30–36.

3. Morrison, M., Murphy, T., and Nalder, C. "Consumer preferences for general practitioner services." *Health Marketing Quarterly* 20 (2004): p. 3–19.

The Journey Begins

Hospital Accreditation Standards and Recommended Practices

Many organizations provide guidelines, standards, and recommendations that are designed to improve patient safety throughout the healthcare system. Several, such as the Joint Commission standards, are well-known among healthcare providers because most hospitals are subject to a Joint Commission accreditation survey roughly every three years (every 18 to 39 months), and nurse managers and directors often must "scramble" to prepare for an imminent survey. But, in addition to Joint Commission standards, there are several other standards and recommendations that are equally important and also represent best practices for improving patient safety. Patient education managers need to be familiar with all of these standards and recommendations and how they affect patient education practices, both directly and indirectly.

Understanding The Joint Commission

The Joint Commission is a private-sector, nonprofit organization that evaluates and assesses healthcare organizations' compliance both with federal regulations and with its own standards. The Joint Commission's published mission is: *"To continuously improve the safety and quality of care provided to the public through the provision of health care accreditation and related services that support performance improvement in health care organizations."*[4] Joint Commission accreditation is directly linked to the Medicare/Medicaid program, because if you meet Joint Commission accreditation standards, you also meet the Medicare *Conditions of Participation,* which is a requirement for receiving Medicare reimbursement from the federal government. This is referred to as "deemed status," meaning that if a hospital meets Joint Commission standards, it is deemed to meet Centers for Medicare & Medicaid Services regulations as well. Despite this direct link to Medicare/Medicaid, The Joint Commission remains an independent, private-sector entity.

Receiving and maintaining Joint Commission accreditation is of utmost importance to hospital administrators and senior executives of healthcare organizations. Therefore, understanding the role The Joint Commission plays in patient education is important in determining the overall landscape of patient education in your healthcare organization. It is critical that every patient education manager is well versed in the Joint Commission standards, as well as in National Patient Safety Goal (NPSG) implications.

The Joint Commission addresses the importance of patient education in several of its standards and National Patient Safety Goals. These standards and goals serve as guidelines to high-quality healthcare. By no means, however, should organizations aspire to meet these standards and goals simply because The Joint Commission requires it; rather, they should do so because the standards and goals are evidence-based and encourage high-quality and safe care to patients. Basically, meeting the standards and goals is the right thing to do.

In 2008, three standards in the *Comprehensive Accreditation Manual for Hospitals* were intended specifically for patient education. Two of the standards, which appear in the Provision of Care chapter, address the need for patients to receive education that is appropriate to both their needs (PC.6.10) and their abilities (PC.6.30). The third standard, which appears in the Leadership chapter, requires leaders to support patient education initiatives and programming (LD.3.120).

In 2009, the standards were revised under the Standards Improvement Initiative, and those revisions included a few changes relative to standards PC.6.10, PC.6.30, and LD.3.120. Essentially, standards PC.6.10 and PC.6.30 were combined to form one standard (PC.02.03.01) that addresses that patient needs *and* abilities are attended to when providing patient education. In addition, standard PC.04.01.05 was added, which requires the organization to provide specific discharge instructions to patients in the event of a discharge or transfer, and to educate patients and their families about any and all follow-up care, treatment, and services.

It's important to note that LD.3.120 was not replicated in the 2009 manual; patient education accountability specifically in the Leadership chapter was deleted. The implications of this are significant; in short, it means that more responsibility is placed on the patient education manager to keep patient education on the radars of senior leadership, through frequent and ongoing communication, demonstrated outcomes, and improvement initiatives. Unfortunately, this often happens only after the organization receives a requirement for improvement (RFI) related to patient education. This is why it is important to devise a proactive and anticipatory approach to identifying potential problem areas for your organization, and to begin to work on action plans to address them. You can do this by ensuring an overall state of survey readiness in your organization.

In my experience, the term *survey readiness* often connotes negativity, because staff members get a sense that we are looking to implement these practices or improvements only to meet Joint Commission requirements. The "scrambling" often seen within organizations when they are preparing for an imminent survey can be exhausting for staff members. And honestly, it does not have to be that way.

We were able to change the way our organization handles survey readiness by taking a different approach. In the past, our centralized education department was responsible for initiating education across the system months before a survey was due. So, for example, a few months before The Joint Commission arrived, we would begin to put up posters and flyers and send e-mails highlighting patient education documentation and the importance of including discharge instructions for all patients. However, though our staff members were able to present well to surveyors, we noticed that they were unable to retrieve information from the electronic medical records (EMR), and thus it appeared that our continuity of care was weak.

In addition, our compliance with patient education documentation was also noted as being very weak. After we addressed these gaps, we worked to have a constant state of readiness in our organization by implementing tracer tools. These tools (see Figure 1.1) follow the Joint Commission tracer methodology and help staff members walk through what is expected of them from a Joint Commission survey perspective. In addition, the tools familiarize the staff members with the EMR and where to retrieve information in an efficient manner. It was surprising to learn that staff members had difficulty retrieving information, such as recent labs, results, progress notes from other care providers, and care plans. Although this could be the result of a particular EMR and its interface, anecdotal information from other organizations seems to suggest this is a common problem.

The tracer tool also proved to have a dual purpose. It not only assisted bedside staff members in being prepared for a survey, but also provided valuable data that could foreshadow problem areas in meeting Joint Commission standards, and thus allowed us to implement more proactive action planning. From this tracer tool, we identified gaps in patient education documentation, indicating that documentation was at 60% compliance.

Inpatient tracer tool

Inpatient Tracer Tool

Department:
Staff Participants:
Patient label:

Date done: / /
Done by:

For each of the items listed below Indicate a Yes if compliant, No if non compliant and NA if not applicable for this patient

Item #	Score Y, N, NA	Description	Item #	Score Y, N, NA	Description
		Ethics, Rights and Responsibilities			**Reassessment**
1		How do you give and where is the patients information about their rights (Patients receive information about their rights) – *staff members be able to state how they provide this information to the patient*	25		Patients are reassessed per policy-systems review (detailed observations and monitoring of systems related to the chief complaint or change in clinical status is present)
2		Hospital general consent form is completed	26		Fall risk - daily
3		Surgical/procedural consent is documented by the MD	27		Skin risk - daily
4		Advance directive information is documented	28		Summary note for each shift - Unit scope document for frequency Days PMs Nights
5		A copy of the advance directive is on the chart	29		Patient is reassessed after PRN or timed pain medication for effect.
6		End of life discussions are documented by the physician	30		Specific to population on unit (neruo, sheaths, Peds...)
7		DNR orders are written on admission			**Development of a plan of care**
		Provision of Care, Treatment & Services	31		Begun on admission
		Initial admission assessments	32		Appropriate for the patient (i.e. high risk areas from HIP – fall, pain, nutrition, skin, functional screen or disease process)
8		Health Information profile is completed/updated on admission - See Policy Standards of clinical practice	33		Individualize to the patients needs
9		Abuse screening is completed within 24 hours of admission	34		Multidisciplinary
10		Nutrition screen completed within 24 hours of admission	35		Short and long term goals are established
11		Functional screen is completed within 24 hours of admission	36		Plan and goals are revised when necessary
12		Past Pain history is assessed on admission	37		Involves the patient/family, significant others as appropriate
13		Current Pain level (intensity) is assessed on admission			**Patient Education Documented as appropriate on the Education Flowsheet** — *Patient is educated about the following*
14		Medication reconciliation is completed on admission. 1. Physician (or RN as telephone order) used Med Reconciliation report to order patient home medications and signed **or** 2. Med Reconciliation report not used for orders, but RN signed on the Medications Reconciled "By line" to indicate that both lists(MDs orders to meds taken at home list in icare) were compared.	38		On the plan for care, treatment and services (they will be receiving)
15		A handwritten H & P/admit note is completed on admission	39		Basic health practices and safety (i.e. call light, bed check, wash hands, bed alarm, bed low position, smoking, vaccine, home environment)
16		Physician admit H & P is dictated, transcribed and authenticated within 24 hours of admission (need all 3)	40		Safe and effective use of medications (Does the patient understand the use of a medication - 1st dose)
17/18		RN initial assessment (systems review) is completed within 8 hours of admission	41		All new medications started in the hospital (reason for, effects, side effects)

Effectively Managed Patient Education

FIGURE 1.1

Inpatient tracer tool (cont.)

Item #	Score Y, N, NA	Description
18		
19		Fall risk assessment (Morris Scale) on admission
20		Aspiration risk assessment on admission
21		Skin assessment (Branden Scale) on admission
22		DVT risk assessment on admission – Start in May
57		Critical test result notification of MD note in summary note (Summary note includes what the value is, interventions received, time of call to the physician) Notification of physician within 30 minutes of critical test result received.
23	x	Specific to population on unit
24	x	Specific to population on unit

Item #	Score Y, N, NA	Description
Discharge planning/instructions		
49		Discharge instructions on activity at home
50		Discharge instructions on when to call the physician
51		Discharge instructions on diet at home
52		Discharge instructions on what to watch for
53		Discharge instructions special monitoring at home (wt. Temp, bleeding, infection, etc.)
54		Medication reconciliation list of take home meds
55		Are written in a form patients can understand
National Patient Safety Goals		
56		Do not use abbreviations are found in the MR (Indicate how many and which one on comment page)
57		Critical test result notification of MD note in summary note Lab result, x-ray.......
58		The surgical/procedural site is marked
59		Final team time out is conducted and documented
60		Medication Reconciliation is done when the patient is transferred in-house to a different level of are
61		On discharge a complete list of meds is given to the next provider of care

Item #	Score Y, N, NA	Description
42		Nutrition, diet or oral health (brush teeth, change in diet....)
43		Safe use of medical equipment and/or medical supplies (any medical equipment used for patient care, discharge equipment to be used)
44		How to obtain further care or treatment if indicated (usually on discharge forms or summary note)
45		Understanding pain, pain management, and methods of assessment
46		Rehabilitation techniques (PT/OT/Speech/CR/Pulm Rehab)
47		Multidisciplinary patient education (PT/RT/Dietary/Pharmacy/OT/CR)
48		Comprehension is assessed on teaching
49		Dietary/Nutrition/Oral health (diet type, eating certain types of nutrient, brushing teeth, dental care)

Item #	Score Y, N, NA	Description
Management of Information		
64		All handwritten orders are dated and timed (Indicate % compliance on Page 3)
65		All handwritten progress notes are dated and timed (Indicate % compliance on Page 3)
66 a.		Handwritten entries are legible a. MD
66b.		b. RNs/Others
67		Medication orders - Name of the medication not abbreviated (Indicate % compliance on Page 3)
68		Progress notes use few /common abbreviations so that the entire care team are aware of the notes meaning and intent.
69		All signatures in the record have name and title
70		Ambulatory areas-problem list/summary list is complete by the 3rd visit
Medication		
71		
72		
73		
74		
75		
76		

Questions to ponder when doing a tracer:

FIGURE 1.1 | Inpatient tracer tool (cont.)

Where would you report a near miss or a potential safety risk?

Describe the pain process for the facility.
Answer: **Admission**
Pain level (intensity) is assessed upon admission or outpatient visit
Pain history is assessed – worst pain experienced and effective interventions
Pain teaching is provided on the pain scale
- *Pain teaching on the pain scale and resources given are documented in the educational flow sheet*
- *Patient level of understanding based upon the teach back method (Rating 0-4)*

Patient's pain goal is documented as appropriate (esp. chronic pain)
Scales utilized are: 0-10, Wong, behavior.
If the patient is able to use the numeric 0-10 then that is the preferred scale
Ongoing
Pain level is assessed with the nursing assessment (based upon unit scope) and by other disciplines (PT, RT)
Prior to giving pain medication the level is assessed with descriptors- location, severity, and quality
Pain medication is given
Patient is taught about the pain medication - reason for, effects, and side effects
- *Pain teaching on the pain medication and resources given are documented in the educational flow sheet*
- *Patient level of understanding based upon the teach back method (Rating 0-4)*

Pain is reassessed after medication is given
Alterative pain relief measures are utilized and documented. (Repositioning, splinting, heat, cold…)

The Joint Commission is on your unit and wants to talk to you about your patient what do you do?
Answer: 1. Communicate to another nurse the needs of the patients you are talking care of
        2. Ask for other disciplines that have been on involved in your patients care to join you with the Joint Commission – dietary, pharmacy, case management, physical therapy….
        3. These other disciplines can assist in answering questions that are specific to the patient and to the process of the coordinated care.

Where would you go to locate what steps to take for a Code White?
Answer: Code White = Emergency Preparedness Plan/Disaster Plan …. Quick reference Safety Flip Chart Located in the department

Locate the Policy on "Standards of Clinical Practice"
Answer: Find policy on line.

What is the value of the above policy to you the bedside nurse?
Answer: Guide for the nursing care provided to patients.   (Assessment, Plan, Intervention, Evaluation)

Comments/ Corrective Action Plan:

Effectively Managing Patient Education

Addressing the gaps in patient education is a challenge, in part because ultimately, accountability for documentation of patient education rests with the organization's bedside care staff. Patient education managers, although often the driving force behind patient education standards and mapping the direction an organization needs to take, lack the ability to truly enforce documentation standards. To address this, organizations need to put in place certain tactics that strengthen the standards and further drive accountability to the bedside staff and their reporting manager. Often, this comes in the form of a corrective action plan.

For example, our corrective action plan (see Figure 1.2) hypothesized what was causing our lack of documentation. By partnering with the quality department, both the information systems and human resources departments developed tactics to address our identified gaps. Including patient education in annual performance reviews and creating documentation standards and specific policies can provide more assurance that patient education documentation will be addressed. By including patient education documentation in performance reviews, you not only underscore patient education's importance in a bedside care role, but also reinforce the idea that patient education documentation is an expectation, since staff members are evaluated based on meeting this requirement. This also places accountability where it belongs: with staff members and their reporting manager. A patient education policy is shown in Figure 1.3.

FIGURE 1.2

Corrective action plan for patient and family education documentation

Problem:

Inpatient tracer cumulative compliance report demonstrates inadequate compliance with all elements of performance of Joint Commission standard PC.02.03.01: *The patient is educated and trained specific to the patient's needs and as appropriate to the care, and services provided.*

Hypothesis:

- Lack of patient education documentation standards and guidelines allow for variability in documentation (content and location).
- Staff perception of patient and family education as a task, rather than ongoing and continuous (i.e.: done but not documented).

Corrective Plan:

Establishment of Patient and Family Education Documentation Guidelines, Education and Accountability

WHAT	Practice Standards	Staff Education	Accountability	Technical Infrastructure
ACTION STEPS	1) Policy development Documentation on flow sheet *only* "Essential elements" of a patient ed interaction 2) Addition of education to daily rounding as applicable 3) Addition of education in shift-to-shift reporting 4) Exploration of processes in place to help with check/balance of patient education (ie: infection control)	Education about new practice standards Education about patient education best practice (i.e.: "teach back," etc)	Addition of patient and family education in staff performance reviews	New education flow sheet pilot
WHO	Nursing Practice Council	Central Education	Managers/directors	IS
WHEN	Within 45 days			July 13th
NOTES	Quality Council to monitor compliance			Pilot estimated to be favorable; will then implement house-wide.

Effectively Managing Patient Education

FIGURE 1.3

Patient and family education
policy and procedure

TITLE:		SECTION: Patient Care

POLICY #:

ORIGIN/DEPARTMENT: Center for Learning and Innovation

EFFECTIVE DATE:

REVIEWED DATE:

	NAME	INITIALS	POSITION	DATE
Prepared By:			Patient Education Coordinator	
Reviewed By:			Executive VP/Chief Nursing Officer	
Reviewed By:			VP/Chief Nursing Executive	
Approved By:			President/CEO	

I. PURPOSE:

To provide guidelines and standardization in the process for patient and family education delivery and documentation.

II. POLICY:

A. It is the responsibility of all healthcare providers to provide patient and family education that will foster patient self-management, promote patient safety and achieve the desired state of wellness as defined in partnership with the patient/family and care providers.

B. Utilizing the Patient Education Process, in partnership with patients/families and the multidisciplinary care team, the healthcare provider shall:

1. Conduct a thorough **education assessment** taking into consideration: patient/family education priorities, health literacy and other language barriers, cultural and religious practices, emotional barriers, drive and motivation to learn, physical and cognitive limitations, and financial implications of care choices.
2. **Plan** educational interventions and identify individualized learning goals, utilizing the data gathered in the assessment.
3. **Teach** utilizing approved patient education materials (handouts, TIGR On-Demand, etc) based upon the patient/family learning preference. Patient education materials should supplement teaching, not replace it.
4. **Evaluate** patient and family understanding of the new knowledge or skill utilizing the "teach-back" method of evaluation.

C. In addition to individualized learning goals, all patients and/or family members shall be educated about:

1. The plan of care, treatment, and services
2. Patient rights and responsibilities
3. Basic health practices and safety

FIGURE 1.3

FIGURE 1.3

Patient and family education policy and procedure (cont.)

4. The safe and effective use of medications
5. Nutrition interventions, modified diets or oral health
6. Safe and effective use of medical equipment or supplies when provided by the hospital
7. Understanding pain, the risk for pain, the importance of effective pain management, the pain assessment process and methods for pain management
8. Habilitation or rehabilitation techniques to help them reach the maximum independence possible.

III. PROCEDURE:

A. All patient and family education, including narrative notes, will be documented in the Patient Education Flow Sheet in the medical record, to allow for care coordination and interdisciplinary collaboration. Patient and family education goals shall be documented in the Care Plan.

B. Patient Education documentation shall include the following **essential elements:**

1. What was taught (i.e: new medication, indication, side effects)
2. What patient education materials were used (i.e: handout)
3. What additional follow-up instruction the patient/family may need

C. Discharge instructions will be completed and given to the patient and/or family prior to discharge. All discharge instructions shall include, but not be limited to, the following:

1. Activity
2. Diet
3. Medications
4. Follow-up appointments
5 When to call the doctor

REFERENCES:
National Quality Forum (2006). Safe Practices for Better Healthcare.

Redman, B. (2006) *The Practice of Patient Education.* **Mosby.**

The 2009 National Patient Safety Goals

The National Patient Safety Goals issued by The Joint Commission are requirements of care that all healthcare organizations must implement and be evaluated on during each accreditation survey. The Joint Commission reviews and updates the Goals annually, amending existing goals or adding others based on new initiatives or evidence. When the Goals were first implemented January 1, 2003, there were just six of them. Today, there are 16 Goals, with various elements of performance for each one. The Universal Protocol™ to prevent wrong-site surgery is also a part of the National Patient Safety Goals.

The Goals were originally developed by the Sentinel Event Alert Advisory Group, a nationally recognized panel of experts comprising pharmacists, physicians, nurses, and other patient safety experts. The Advisory Group first convened in April 2002 and developed recommendations after reviewing The Joint Commission's *Sentinel Event Alerts*.[5] From those alerts, the Advisory Group identified 44 recommendations that potentially might have a great effect in improving patient safety in hospitals across the nation. Of those 44 recommendations, the Advisory Group prioritized and presented their top six recommendations to The Joint Commission's Board of Commissioners. Those recommendations were approved, and were implemented nationwide in 2003.[5] The Advisory Group, now called the Patient Safety Advisory Group, continues to review the Goals annually and identifies upcoming topics for both future goal development and *Sentinel Event Alert* publications.

The first six Goals were announced in July 2002, and they were widely accepted by many practitioners, as they were topics that had been in discussion for many years. The Goals are evidence-based and extremely cost-effective, with practical strategies for implementation.[4]

The Goals are designed to keep patients safe; they focus on problematic areas in healthcare and offer solutions to help resolve them. The solutions are generally system-focused in an effort to recognize that a truly safe environment is one that operates as seamlessly as possible. The Goals include all aspects of care, ranging from how to safely identify a patient before a procedure, to hand hygiene and central line infections.

Of particular importance is the role that patient education plays in these Goals. The 2009 National Patient Safety Goals have expanded to include more detailed Elements of Performance for certain Goals, with significant patient education or patient–provider communication implications for many of them. See Figure 1.4 for a list of the NPSGs that relate to patient education.

FIGURE 1.4 — The 2009 National Patient Safety Goals and their corresponding Elements of Performance

2009 National Patient Safety Goal	2009 Element of Performance Expansion
Goal #3: Safe medication usage	Patients and their families are educated on standardized anticoagulants.
Goal #7: Decreased healthcare-associated infections	Patients and their families are educated on standardized multidrug-resistant organisms.
Goal #8: Medication reconciliation	Patients and their families are educated on their medication lists.
Goal #13: Patient involvement in care	Patients and their families understand that specific safety measures are evaluated and documented.

The National Quality Forum

The National Quality Forum (NQF), established in 1999, is a private, nonprofit organization whose purpose is to develop a national strategy for healthcare quality measurement and reporting. The NQF is composed of many organizations from all parts of the healthcare system, including consumers, employers, healthcare professionals, provider organizations, health plans, accrediting bodies, and labor unions. The group formed with a shared concern over healthcare quality and its effect on patient outcomes, patient safety, productivity, and rising healthcare costs. The NQF's mission statement, published on its Web site, reads as follows: "To improve the quality of American healthcare by setting national priorities and goals for performance improvement, endorsing national consensus standards for measuring and publicly reporting on performance, and promoting the attainment of national goals through education and outreach programs."[6] In addition, the NQF's vision, taken from the NQF Web site, reads as follows:

- *The NQF will be the convener of key public and private sector leaders to establish national priorities and goals to achieve the Institute of Medicine Aims—healthcare that is safe, effective, patient-centered, timely, efficient, and equitable*

- *NQF-endorsed standards will be the primary standards used to measure and report on the quality and efficiency of healthcare in the United States*

- *The NQF will be recognized as a major driving force for, and facilitator of, continuous quality improvement of American healthcare quality*[15]

 Effectively Managing Patient Education

The NQF endorsed 30 Safe Practices in 2003 that should be "universally utilized in applicable clinical care settings to reduce the risk of error and resultant harm to patients,"[16] recognizing the healthcare safety movement that by this point had become a national priority. Each of the Safe Practices, updated in 2006 and again in 2009 to include a total of 34, is specific, easily generalized, and evidence-based, ready to be implemented. Patient education managers need to be familiar with these Safe Practices, as a few of them directly involve patient education. All Safe Practices are organized into the following categories:[7]

- Creating and sustaining a culture of safety

- Informed consent, honoring patient wishes, and disclosure

- Matching healthcare needs with service delivery capability

- Medication management

- Preventing healthcare-associated infections

- Condition- and site-specific practices

It's important to note that the NQF intentionally does not prioritize or weight any of these practices, as each is considered to be equally important to implement. Each is critical to ensuring patients are kept safe.

Practices for creating and sustaining a culture of safety, although not as directly linked to patient education as in the Safe Practices, are important for everyone to follow, as doing so helps to meet an end goal which every department shares: patient safety. In my organization, we utilized a Culture of Patient Safety Toolkit that helped clinical managers prepare their bedside staff in creating and sustaining a culture of safety. This toolkit, located in Appendix Three of this book, was available for managers to use as activities during staff meetings or departmental inservices, since it is often a challenge to get staff members away from the bedside for any type of extensive education. This approach was successful for us in that it provided a resource to unit managers who were often in the best position to transfer information to the staff.

Of particular importance to patient education are practices that directly affect patient education. Safe Practice #2, under the broader category of Informed Consent, speaks to how practitioners need to assess comprehension, once instruction has been given, by utilizing the "teach-back" method. This method involves asking patients and/or family members to restate in their own words key information about what they learned or were told regarding any treatments or procedures for which they need to give informed consent.

Although the teach-back method is recommended as a Safe Practice during the informed consent process, organizations should use this method for *any* patient education interaction, as it truly is an effective way to evaluate what the patient comprehends. You should avoid asking the classic question, "Do you understand?" as patients will rarely want to disclose that they didn't understand, or they may not even be aware of any knowledge gap.[8] Rather, reframing the question—as in, "Tell me what you're going to tell your friends and family about how to manage your disease at home," or "I want to make sure I taught you everything you need to know, so to help me know that I did that, explain to me how you would take your medication"—is a much better approach that will truly assess what the patient learned from the instruction. In addition, as related to consent, the patient will truly be able to provide informed consent, and staff members will have assurances that the patient is fully informed about his or her procedure and its risks and benefits.

Another Safe Practice recommends that the organization ensures that information is communicated to patients in a "clearly understandable form."[16] This means all aspects of communication with patients and their families, from verbal interactions to written handouts, are clear. But what does it mean to be "clearly understandable"? To be clearly understandable, information must be communicated in such a way that the receiver understands the message you are trying to convey.

The Plain Language Movement in the U.S. government is a perfect example of why this is necessary and how to go about speaking and writing in "plain language." Plain language has been addressed at the government level in the United States since before the 1970s, starting with a publication called *Gobbledygook Has Got to Go*.[9] From there, various initiatives throughout government have transpired. Plain language gained lots of momentum during the Clinton Administration, when Vice President Al Gore considered communications in plain language to be a civil right, and a practice that promotes trust in the government. In fact, the U.S. Securities and Exchange Commission's (SEC) *A Plain English Handbook* remains a perfect example of a document that is written in plain language. Warren Buffett, a friend of the SEC chairman at the time the handbook was published, offered this definition of writing in plain language:

> *Write with a specific person in mind. When writing the Berkshire Hathaway annual report, I picture my sisters, highly intelligent, but not experts in accounting or finance. They will understand plain English, but jargon may puzzle them. My goal is to give the information I would wish to receive if our positions were reversed.*[9]

Clearly, communications from our federal government are important enough that all people should understand them; the same is true with healthcare. When speaking to a patient and his or her family about a new diagnosis or treatment the patient must undergo, or when writing and designing a handout that will be given to patients, consider Warren Buffett's definition. More tips on how to prepare reader-friendly patient education handouts will appear later in the book.

Culturally and Linguistically Appropriate Services (CLAS) standards

The Office of Minority Health (OMH) developed the Culturally and Linguistically Appropriate Services (CLAS) standards in response to growing concern regarding the healthcare needs of minorities. The standards were developed by analyzing existing laws and standards, and were further refined by several project committees, with the aim of ensuring culturally appropriate care and cultural competence. The emergence of cultural competence as a method to close the gap in racial and ethnic disparities in healthcare[10] came about due to the ever-increasing diversity of the United States. The goal of cultural competency is "to create a health care system and workforce that are capable of delivering the highest-quality care to every patient regardless of race, ethnicity, culture, or language proficiency."[10] Nurses and other healthcare professionals are faced with a global population, with varying beliefs, languages, and approaches to medicine. As a result, staff members need to be well-versed in how to provide care to patients with such diversity.

The OMH, a function of the U.S. Department of Health and Human Services, exists to develop health policies, programs, and standards to close ethnic and racial gaps in healthcare and to ensure that all minorities receive the care they need in order to stay healthy. As a result, the OMH developed the CLAS standards to assist hospitals in providing culturally and linguistically appropriate care. There are 14 standards, grouped by theme and falling under one of three stringencies: mandates, guidelines, or recommendations. Those that are deemed mandates are required actions by healthcare entities in order to receive federal funding.[21] The themes in which the standards fall are: Culturally Competent Care (Standards 1–3), Language Access Services (Standards 4–7), and Organizational Supports for Cultural Competence (Standards 8–14). Of particular relevance to patient education is Standard 7 (a mandate), which speaks to how patient education materials not only must be easily understood, but also must be available in the patient's language. So, if your hospital commonly sees Spanish-speaking patients, you are obligated to ensure that your materials are also provided in Spanish. We will discuss culturally appropriate care and patient education in more detail later in this book.

The guidance in Standard 7 is as follows:

> *Healthcare organizations must make available easily understood patient-related mate-*
> *rials and post signage in the languages of the commonly encountered groups and/or*
> *groups represented in the service area.*[11]

The Institute for Healthcare Improvement (IHI)

The Institute for Healthcare Improvement (IHI) is an independent, nonprofit organization dedicated to improving healthcare quality via various initiatives aimed at improving patient safety worldwide. By recommending key initiatives, building energy and enthusiasm to change, and providing resources for hospitals to deploy the initiatives, the IHI hopes to accomplish the following:[12]

- No needless deaths

- No needless pain or suffering

- No helplessness in those served or serving

- No unwanted waiting

- No waste

- No one left out

Two of the largest improvement initiatives in healthcare are the IHI's *100,000 Lives Campaign* and *5 Million Lives Campaign*, in which recommendations for saving patients from harm in one year's time are shared and hospitals are called to action to participate. Each year since the inception of those initiatives, the IHI has added new recommendations and renewed energy. Thus far, patient education has had an indirect link to the IHI's initiatives; however, it's still important to stay abreast of what the IHI recommends each year. In late 2008, the IHI launched its newest campaign, *The Improvement Map*, which will focus on improving 100 processes within hospitals vital to great patient care.

Reviewing the literature

As with other clinical questions of inquiry, knowing "what's happening" in the world of patient education is a must. This starts with a comprehensive literature review. Many librarians can assist you in this endeavor; however, knowing how to search on your own is a good skill to have. Many resources are available to help you learn how to search through databases and decipher literature findings; among the most helpful resources is *Essentials of Nursing Research: Methods, Appraisal and Utilization,* by Denise F. Polit and Cheryl Tatano Beck (Lippincott).

 Effectively Managing Patient Education

There are many reasons to conduct a literature review. For the purposes of managing patient education at the organizational level, it means analyzing study findings and assessing their applicability to your organization, determining any implications they may have, and developing subsequent recommendations. The literature can hold answers to these and many other questions regarding patient education:

- If your organization lacks a policy on patient education materials, how do you know what your policy statement should cover?

- What is a best practice on material development?

- What is the best way to measure comprehension after a teaching interaction?

- What are other organizations doing and what are some lessons learned?

Conducting a literature review will help guide your next steps, and also helps to ensure that your methods are best practices. In addition, the following resources are invaluable to new patient education managers and are considered a core collection for staying up to date and well-informed:

Journals

Patient Education & Counseling (Elsevier)

Patient Education Management (AHC Media)

Books

The Joint Commission Guide to Patient and Family Education (Joint Commission Resources)

Teaching Patients with Low Literacy Skills by Celia C. Doak, Leonard G. Doak, and Jane H. Root (Lippincott)

No Time to Teach? by Fran London (Lippincott)

The Practice of Patient Education by Barbara Klug Redman (Mosby)

Patient Education: Principles & Practice by Sally H. Rankin and Karen Duffy Stallings (Lippincott)

The Illness Narratives: Suffering, Healing & the Human Condition by Arthur Kleinman (Basic Books)

Understanding Health Literacy: Implications for Medicine and Public Health (American Medical Association)

Crucial Conversations: Tools for Talking When the Stakes Are High by Kerry Patterson, Joseph Grenny, Ron McMillan, et al. (McGraw Hill)

Radical Loving Care: Building the Healing Hospital in America by Erie Chapman (Baptist Health Healing Trust)

Web sites

www.jointcommission.org

www.thecommonwealthfund.org

www.healthliteracy.com

www.ahrq.gov

Professional organizations

Health Care Education Association

Assessing the environment

When you begin your career in patient education management, analyze your organization and collect some data to get a better understanding of the overall landscape. You need not be a statistician to collect data. Data can come from any number of avenues, both quantitative and qualitative in nature. Data can mean anything, from the number of patient education materials you have in foreign languages to dollars spent on patient education. Some topics lend themselves well to data collection; for example, if your facility has an on-demand patient education video system, you may be able to easily determine the usage rate of any and all patient education videos in your organization. Asking questions and knowing where your organization stands regarding patient education will help to guide your efforts and prioritize your energy. Use the following questions to understand the current state of patient education in your organization:

• How is patient education delivered?

• Are any competencies related to patient education?

- Are the patient education materials of high quality? Do they require only a low reading level?

- Is patient education documented appropriately?

- Is your organization meeting Joint Commission standards?

- What do clinical staff members think of the current state of patient education? Are their needs met?

- What does your chief nursing officer think is the greatest priority?

Suppose the answers to the preceding questions reveal the following: patient education appears to be delivered primarily via the nursing staff through handouts and verbal instruction. Usage of education videos is low to nonexistent, and the videos that are in the facility are more than 10 years old. There aren't any competencies for patient education; documentation, however, appears to be good and your organization is Joint Commission–accredited and had minimal RFIs at the last survey. The staff thinks patient education overall is "fine," but the chief nursing officer believes the staff is lacking basic skills in educating patients and shows you patient satisfaction reports that support this claim. What area would you focus on first? What would be your recommendation for action?

These findings, combined with the latest trends found in the literature, will provide valuable insights. Use the data gathered, as well as your interpretation of the data and subsequent recommendations, to prepare a formal assessment report. Collecting this data, preparing the report, and communicating your findings to senior leaders in your organization will assist in the buy-in process, particularly if you are looking for additional funding, full-time equivalent support, or expansion of existing services.

In many cases, only a quick "glance" by a patient education manager will reveal that improvement is required in all areas of patient education. Chart audits might reveal inconsistent charting with missing elements; comprehension is assessed via the classic "Do you understand?" and was validated by a patient's signature on discharge instructions. Materials handed out to patients might lack unity and clarity and are decentralized in a way that costs the organization far more than it should. Resources for patients range from limited to nonexistent.

More likely than not, *several* areas need attention and organization. But you can't change all of them at once. Keep in mind that too much change all at once can lead to "repetitive-change syndrome," which can mean initiative overload, change-related chaos, and widespread employee anxiety, cynicism, and burnout.[13] To ensure that your changes are met with the least amount of resistance, find the *one area* that needs the most improvement and whose resolution would have the most effect; garner support for that first, and resolve that issue. And do it well.

Navigating Through the Change Process

Change is hard, and even harder to manage on your own. In fact, in organizations the world over, many change efforts fail before they even begin to take hold. Why? First, it's important to recognize that any amount of change requires several phases that, in total, equal a large amount of time. Even though the change needed may be urgent or may seem relatively easy to execute, for the change to take hold and become part of the everyday business or culture in your organization, you need to invest in *time*.

Finding that one area to focus on and change for the better can be overwhelming. How do you decide? If you're a patient education manager, everything about patient education is a priority. The reality, however, is that it can't all be done at once; and if you're new to the organization, you don't want to come on board proposing sweeping changes. Instead, several great tools are available to help you prioritize your needs.

One such tool is the priority/payoff matrix (see Figure 1.5). You can use this tool to analyze an option from two different angles. If the issue falls into the "high payoff" and "easy to implement" categories, it is reasonable to infer that this is the issue toward which you should prioritize your efforts. In our organization, after we determined our current status through data collection and a subsequent assessment report, we placed problem areas on the payoff matrix. Actually deciding where something falls in the matrix often requires discussion and a group consensus. We identified several areas in patient education to work on, but on our payoff matrix, improving the education flow sheet for easier documentation in our EMR was believed to be "high priority/easy to implement." "Easy," of course, was relative, since we also had to partner with our information systems department to make this happen. But the payoff matrix proved to be a useful tool; we focused our energy on improving and implementing the flow sheet, and our caregivers' perception of the usefulness of education documentation improved by 30% within two months.

 Effectively Managing Patient Education

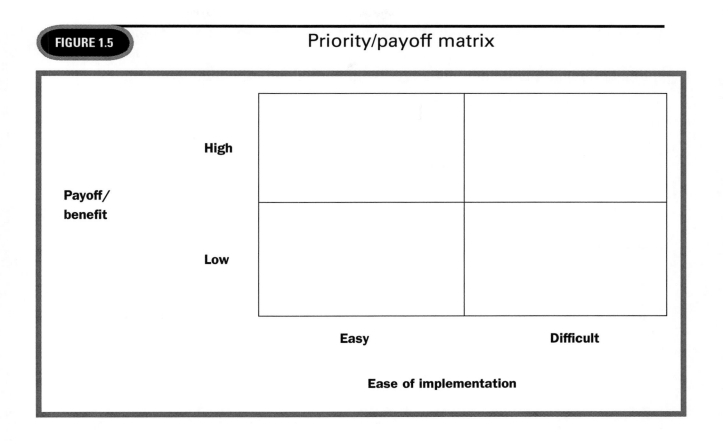

FIGURE 1.5 Priority/payoff matrix

Once you've identified the high-priority/easy-to-implement tactic you should work on, be cognizant of the change process and what it takes to create and roll out a successful change. John P. Kotter, a Harvard Business School faculty member who is highly regarded as the foremost authority on change, change management, and leadership, outlines eight crucial factors in managing change in his work, *Leading Change* (Harvard Business School Press). Understanding each factor is an important skill for any patient education manager to have, and is crucial to ensuring a successful transformation.

Factor 1: Establish a sense of urgency

It's hard to implement a major transformational change when nobody in your organization believes there is reason to change in the first place. Getting people to buy into the need to change means demonstrating to them why change is needed. Literature reviews, benchmarking data, and competitor analysis are all valuable pieces of information that can lead to establishing a shared need to change. But it's also important to include what will happen *if change does not occur*. For patient education programs, it could mean revenue loss, Joint Commission citations, a decrease in patient satisfaction scores, liability to the organization, or, worse, patient safety risks.

Don't underestimate the amount of effort it may require to get people on board with your proposal. Even though the need for change may exist, getting people to move out of their comfort zone may take more effort than is realized. Often, people may start to tell themselves a story about potential horrible domino effects once a change has taken place, such as morale suffering as a result of new regulations, staff turnover, system problems, and the like. And many times, these concerns may be valid, and you should consider them within the larger context of the proposal. They should not paralyze leaders from taking action, however. Rather, it's important to remember that "change, by definition, requires creating a new system, which in turn always demands leadership."[13]

Factor 2: Create a powerful guiding coalition

As mentioned earlier in this chapter, change is hard to manage, especially alone. For a successful change initiative, having a core group of influential decision-makers guiding the process helps tremendously in ensuring that the change effort sustains over the long term and gains momentum. These influential decision-makers, in the most successful of groups, aren't necessarily all senior executives, but rather are powerful individuals in terms of title, influence, reputation, and relationships.

A critical component is that the coalition has an executive sponsor, or a senior leader who can guide the process, remove barriers, and help foster and support change at the highest level of the organization. In our organization, this person was our integration officer. This was a new executive position designed to help our multi–health facility organization integrate into one system. Since patient education also needed to be integrated throughout the system, this executive seemed like a logical choice. I scheduled an appointment with her to discuss patient education, the current state of the organization, my recommendations, and the need for executive sponsorship.

This approach is also consistent with the experience of a Veterans Administration Medical Center, which found that "a strong linkage to the executive management team was necessary if patient education was to be an integral part of the medical center."[14] Recognizing that any amount of change requires the effort of other people is a critical factor to the success of any recommendation that is being proposed. For many organizations, a good step to take to begin that change process is to establish that guiding coalition with a systemwide patient education committee. Any system-level committee at the leadership level can be costly to the organization in terms of both time and money, so it's important to outline a proposal for this to gain buy-in. Figure 1.6 shows an executive summary from a comprehensive proposal for a system-level committee.

FIGURE 1.6 | **Executive summary from a comprehensive proposal for a system-level committee**

Executive summary

State of affairs

The organization lacks a standard and unified process for the creation, implementation, and distribution of patient education documents and initiatives. Patient education occurs reactively as opposed to proactively, and without any strategic planning.

Although individual patient education documents may be of excellent clinical quality, collectively they lack consistency in the messages they deliver to patients. In addition, the materials given to patients are generally written at the graduate level, and most likely patients are unable to understand them.

The organization also lacks any archival process for its patient education documents. This continually puts the organization at risk because it is unable to determine what education was provided to a patient on any given health topic.

Risks and opportunities

Strengths	Weaknesses
• Organizational willingness to align • Executive support • Many frontline staff members invested in writing materials • "Homegrown" documents; allows for distinct customization	• Consistency • Organizational standards • Budget dollars • Archiving • Community image
Opportunities	**Threats**
• Linkage to the Hospital Consumer Assessment of Healthcare Providers and Systems (HCAHPS): trending in qualitative patient perception of care • Linkage to patient-/family-centered care approach	• Regulatory bodies • Competition most likely will penetrate service area • Patient safety • Litigation • Patient perception

| FIGURE 1.6 | Executive summary from a comprehensive proposal for a system-level committee (cont.) |

Recommendations

1. Form a committee at the executive level (Patient Education Advisory Committee), which will direct and manage patient education activities at an organizational level. A subcommittee comprising expert clinicians (health education review group, or HERG) would serve to operationalize the vision put forth by the patient education advisory committee.

2. Fully implement Ask Me 3 *(www.askme3.org)* at an organizational level.

Budget

The following is a budget proposal for implementation of the patient education advisory committee and the HERG subcommittee. Implementation of Ask Me 3 requires no direct cost.

Direct Salaries and Wages

Personnel

Total: **$16,444.56**

Subtotal for nonmanagement staff: $7,750.80

Subtotal for management staff: $8,693.76

Employees	Average hourly salary	Time per month (two hours)	Months	Amount per resource
Managers and directors for the patient education advisory committee: total of 16 members	$22.64	1.28%	12 months	$543.36
Staff for HERG (nonmanagers/ directors): total of 15 employees	$21.53	1.28%	12 months	$516.72

Strategic goal alignment

Implementation of the recommendations put forth in this assessment is consistent and in alignment with the following two major strategic initiatives:

- Patient-/family-centered care
- Cost and quality

FIGURE 1.6

Executive summary from a comprehensive proposal for a system-level committee (cont.)

Measures of success

Although currently neither national standards nor benchmarking data for patient education exist, you can use several metrics to measure success of patient education:

- Patient satisfaction scores:
  - Press Ganey
  - HCAHPS
- Patient feedback:
  - Focus groups
- Joint Commission standards and Core Measures
- Reading level of patient education documents
- Number of documents in Spanish
- Number of other foreign languages offered
- Online access of all patient education documents
- Consistent patient education document template
- Awards for patient education (National Health Information Awards; *www.healthawards.com/ nhia/details.htm)*

Factor 3: Create a vision

It's been said that one of the major reasons teams fail is the lack of a shared vision; goals may be unclear, leading to an uncoordinated effort that often results in duplicity, confusion, and, eventually, apathy. Creating that shared vision is a crucial first step once a powerful team has been assembled, to be certain that everyone is on track and is moving toward one agreed-upon and measurable goal. Creating a shared vision means coming together as a team with a shared understanding of the need for change, and determining together what the end result will look like.

Later in this book, I will discuss specific tools that will help you to define what that vision is and to map it out within a group. See Figure 1.7 for an example of what a mission, vision, and goals for patient education can look like.

 Effectively Managing Patient Education

FIGURE 1.7 Mission, vision, and goals for patient education, established by the patient education committee

We support patients, families, and the community in their quest for health and well-being by providing quality health education that is informative and individualized. We believe in empowering patients and families, through education, to achieve and maintain health and safety, and encouraging an active partnership between our healthcare providers and the people they serve.

Patient education vision statement:
Providing an interdisciplinary framework for which patient education can be fully integrated throughout the organization and the healthcare continuum.

Goals:

Ongoing:
- Address the learning needs and preferences of people from all literacy levels, populations, and cultures we serve
- Support and promote patient education efforts within the organization
- Provide current, research-based patient and family education
- Utilize an outcome-based approach to patient education

2007–2008 goals:
- Develop and implement a process, along with criteria, for creating patient and family educational materials throughout the organization
- Develop a complete inventory of all current English and Spanish patient and family educational materials throughout the organization
- Develop and maintain an archival process for all patient and family educational materials throughout the organization
- Evaluate inventory of all current patient and family educational materials throughout the organization against the newly created criteria
- Identify additional patient and family education needs and prioritize development
- Identify other cultural language needs for our community
- Identify process for financial support of development and implementation of patient and family educational materials

Factor 4: Communicate!

Kotter notes that "in more successful transformation efforts, executives use all existing communication channels to broadcast the vision."[15] When the vision isn't strongly communicated, and, even more importantly, when leaders in the organization don't model the new behaviors for change, momentum for change can be lost. Developing a comprehensive communication plan in partnership with corporate communications can enhance communication methods and ensure that all intended audiences are reached. See Figure 1.8 for an example of a communication plan.

Suppose, for example, that you are unveiling a new on-demand patient education video system. You decided to obtain this video system after your assessment report reveals that availability of patient education videos is lacking in your organization, and after the payoff matrix reveals that implementing this would bring a high payoff. In addition, it would probably resolve some of your patient satisfaction scores. Unveiling the system is great, but if its availability is not adequately communicated, it won't take hold in the organization, and you will risk a failed implementation.

FIGURE 1.8 — Patient education project: Communication plan

Authors: Patient Education Manager
Corporate Communications Manager
Education Director
Chief Administrative Officer

Overarching communication message:

In support of patient-/family-centered care, our organization will convert to a centralized, single on-line source for patient education throughout the organization starting in March 2009. The goal of this conversion is to provide the organization with a source for clear, consistent, and clinically current healthcare information that is readily available to patients and their families, hospital staff members, and physicians. In addition to improved access to the materials, the online source will enhance collaboration, efficiency, professionalism, flexibility, and comprehensiveness of the information being provided to patients on behalf of our organization. The resource will be available to anyone with a printer and access to the Web.

Audience	Message	Message vehicles	Timing	Responsibility
Physicians, PAs, MD office staff, NPs	Overarching message, plus: Print what you need right in your office via the Web and a centricity link in EMR Links and instructions Resource to contact for live support Conversion to this system is required throughout the organization. There will be an organizationwide effort to purge outdated educational resources by _____ (date).	Physician newsletter Demonstrations and discussions at division meetings, outside of all staff conferences Quick user's guide	4 weeks prior to launch	Corporate editor Patient ed manager Patient ed manager

FIGURE 1.8	Patient education project: Communication plan (cont.)

Audience	Message	Message vehicles	Timing	Responsibility
Leadership	Overarching communication message: This is coming in March. As we are gearing up for the transition, please begin to use this process now to request new materials. Here are the details....	Leader e-mails	Four months prior, once ready to discuss	Communications strategist
		Leader e-mails	Start four weeks prior to launch	Communications strategist
	Overarching message, plus: Your leadership among staff in support of this change is requested, as evidenced by compliance for your area Links and instructions Resource to contact for live support Conversion to this system is required throughout the organization. There will be an organizationwide effort to purge outdated educational resources by _____ (date).	Fact sheet/ talking points Demo to leaders at site leadership meetings Quick user's guide		Communications strategist and patient ed manager Patient ed manager Patient ed manager

Effectively Managing Patient Education

FIGURE 1.8   Patient education project: Communication plan (cont.)

Audience	Message	Message vehicles	Timing	Responsibility
All employees	Overarching communication message: This is coming in March. As we are gearing up for the transition, please begin to use this process now to request new materials. Here are the details....	Huddle Intranet Manager discussion Town halls	June/July as appropriate	Communications strategist
	Overarching message, plus: Print what you need when you need it Links and instructions Resource to contact for live support Conversion to this system is required throughout the organization. There will be an organizationwide effort to purge outdated educational resources by _____ (date).	E-mail campaign, including IS newsletter Huddles Intranet	Start four weeks prior to launch	Communications strategist
Clinical employees	Launch messages, plus more detail about using new resources and procedure for creating new pieces	Training classes (?) Agenda item for key department meetings Quick user's guide	Four weeks prior to launch	Patient ed manager

FIGURE 1.8 Patient education project: Communication plan (cont.)

Audience	Message	Message vehicles	Timing	Responsibility
Patients and families	Overarching message, plus: Resource is available to you and your family members online via easy access on hospital Web sites	Patient user's guide Patient information materials and discharge instructions Consumer Web sites	At launch	Patient ed manager Web strategist

   Effectively Managing Patient Education

Factor 5: Remove obstacles to the vision for patient education

Paradoxically, removing obstacles to the vision can be an obstacle in itself, and it can present the patient education manager with the single largest challenge in the change effort. Sometimes one of the larger, more destructive obstacles can be a key senior leader who is not on board with the change effort and who may actively work against the effort by allowing rogue behaviors to continue. In these cases, particularly when the person is a senior leader and the behavior isn't addressed but is allowed to continue, the entire change effort can collapse. This is where having an executive sponsor who is a senior-level leader can assist to ensure that these barriers are addressed and/or removed.

For example, suppose a senior leader isn't on board with the campaign to rewrite and reformat all of your organization's patient education materials to be at a low reading level for patients, and this senior leader does not support the new process in place for patient education materials to be approved before use. Since this leader isn't on board with the process, neither are the staff members. They continue to write and obtain renegade patient education materials and do not follow the process of having them reviewed or approved. Having such an obstacle in the way can seriously thwart the efforts of your initiative. Once aware of the obstacle, an executive sponsor can have those crucial conversations with that leader and can likely work to remove the barrier on your behalf.

Factor 6: Systematically plan for and create short-term wins

According to Kotter, "most people won't go on the long march unless they see compelling evidence in 12 to 24 months that the journey is producing expected results. Without short term wins, too many people give up or actively join the ranks of those people who have been resisting change."[15] With this in mind, it's important to build in some short-term gains that the staff can celebrate, but by no means should these gains equate to victory. The following represent some short-term wins:

- Mission, vision, and goals were developed and accepted by the executive team

- New processes were established to support the vision

- The organization reached its interim benchmarks

Celebrating these short-term wins demonstrates to the team that progress is being made and their efforts are paying off. Without this, it's easy for the team to feel disillusioned and think they will not meet their ultimate goal.

Factor 7: Do not declare victory too soon

If your organization announces that all the goals have been met before the transformation has had a chance to really be embedded into the culture, there is a high risk that people's initial inertia and passion for the change effort will dwindle and they will return to their normal duties, which in many cases may mean the "old ways." Furthermore, those people who were resistant to the change all along will use the victory celebration as evidence that no further change effort is needed: The battle is over and has been won. The risk is then very high that in two years, the processes that were set up could begin to unravel. In Kotter's experience, he noted that in these cases ". . . the useful changes that had been introduced slowly disappeared. In two of the ten cases, it's hard to find any trace of the reengineering work today."[15] This is why it's important to build in those short-term wins, so people do feel a sense of accomplishment, but also make sure that these wins aren't seen as the final victory celebration.

Factor 8: Anchor changes into the organization's culture

You can ensure that changes are built into the organization's culture in two ways. The first way is to connect the dots for people. When positive results are realized after a change has occurred, often people may associate the results with a new management team, the opening of a new hospital, or some other inaccurate link. You should make a significant effort to connect those dots and communicate how the change effort produced those results. For example, suppose that once patient education materials were reformatted to be patient-centered, patient satisfaction scores rose; there was a notable decrease in call volumes to the call center; and there were fewer readmissions for disease management lapses. Although certainly it could be argued that other factors may have contributed *overall* to these metrics, it is important to make the connection regarding how the patient education change effort influenced these results. Communicate this to staff via meetings, newsletter articles, and other common communication venues. If the connection isn't made for them, they will make it themselves, and most likely it will be inaccurate.

The second way to ensure that changes are built into the organization's culture is to ensure that any successors for senior positions buy into the change effort, so as to not undermine the culture years later when they are in a higher position of authority. Although this particular tactic may seem out of the scope and influence of the patient education manager, recognizing that having a strong, solid connection to senior leadership is crucial to minimizing this risk as much as possible. Establishing the connection to senior leadership happens primarily through ongoing networking. If your organization has quarterly "leadership retreats" or "leadership development institutes" or other types of forums where the organization's leaders come together for a day of learning and development, you need to attend those as well. Not only do those forums provide a great venue for continuing education on various leadership topics, but also they typically provide a way for

                          Effectively Managing Patient Education

people to interact with one another. Relationship-building and networking is a necessity to effectively do your job.

Understanding change and how to manage it in large healthcare organizations is a critical competency for any patient education manager. For patient education to remain a viable and important aspect of the healthcare continuum, patient education managers must advocate and plan for change; they must challenge the status quo and obtain the attention and support of senior-level executives. Once you have those skills, patient education can expand to the next level.

References

4. The Joint Commission. "A Journey Through the History of the Joint Commission." The Joint Commission Web site, *www.jointcommission.org/AboutUs/joint_commission_history.htm* (accessed August 18, 2008).

5. May, Sondra. "National Patient Safety Goals: a new patient safety initiative." *Hospital Pharmacy*, 38 (2003): 490-496.

6. National Quality Forum. "Mission Statement." The National Quality Forum Web site, *http://qualityforum.org/about/mission.asp* (accessed November 6, 2008).

7. National Quality Forum. "Safe Practices for Better Healthcare 2006 Update." *www.qualityforum.org/publications/asp* (accessed November 6, 2008).

8. Youmans, S., and Schillinger, D. "Functional health literacy and the pharmacist's role," *The Annals of Pharmacotherapy* 37 (2003): 1726-9. *www.safetynetinstitute.org/resources/chroniccare/PharmicstRole.pdf* (accessed November 7, 2008).

9. Plain Language. "Improving Communications from the Federal Government to the Public." *www.plainlanguage.gov.* (accessed September 20, 2008).

10. Bentacourt, J., Green, A., Carillo, E., and Park, E. "Cultural competence and health care disparities: key perspectives and trends," *Health Affairs* 24: (2005). *http://content.healthaffairs.org/cgi/content/full/24/2/499* (accessed November 8, 2008).

11. The Office of Minority Health. *www.omhrc.gov/templates/browse.aspx?lvl=2&lvlID=15* (accessed November 8, 2008).

12. Institute for Healthcare Improvement. *www.ihi.org/ihi* (accessed November 8, 2008).

13. Abrahamson, E. *Change Without Pain: How Managers Can Overcome Initiative Overload, Organizational Chaos and Employee Burnout.* Boston: Harvard Business School Press, 2003, p. 3.

14. Cordell, B., Linnel, K., and Price, J. "Strategic planning in patient education: A key element of successful management." *Patient Education and Counseling* 11 (1988): p. 65–73.

15. Kotter, J. "Leading change: Why transformation efforts fail." *Harvard Business Review* (January 2007): p. 96–100.

Obtaining Organizational Support

The Importance of Organizational Support

Where patient education exists within an organization can vary across hospital systems, but generally it has a reporting function that falls within the clinical education department. Because of this, when compared to clinical education, *patient* education is often in a unique position; it's one of the few functions within a support department that has a direct effect on patient care and whose products or outcomes, such as patient education materials, tools, and programs, actually *touch* patients. By contrast, *clinical* education affects patient care more indirectly by providing the support and skills necessary to providers of care to ensure patient safety and care quality.

Patient education does have a logical fit within the hospital's education department by virtue of its shared purpose, which is to educate others; at times, however, this structure can pose additional challenges. In these difficult economic times, when all service industries, particularly nonprofit organizations, are watching their bottom line and must cut expenses, one of the first things to take a cut is funds for education. The reasons for this often stem from a "nice to have" versus "need to have" analysis. When faced with the decision to fund additional full-time equivalents (FTE) to provide direct patient care ("need to have") or to educate the existing staff ("nice to have"), the FTE will win out. Patient education managers must be prepared to advocate for how and why patient and family education services, despite being hidden in a centralized education department, fall in the "need to have" category. Imagine a hospital environment where the following takes place:

- A newly diagnosed diabetic patient is discharged home without being told anything about his diagnosis, how to self-inject insulin, or how to check his blood sugar.

- A new mom gives birth to premature twins at 30 weeks' gestation. The twins are in the NICU for several months and need to be gavage-fed upon going home, as well as monitored with apnea monitors. The twins are discharged home with the necessary equipment (special formula, gavage tube, and monitors), and their parents aren't told a single thing about how to take care of them.

- A 35-year-old female patient is about to undergo a hysterectomy for uterine cancer; however, no one has told the patient why she needed this surgery, or exactly what is being removed and what that means for her.

Can you imagine any of these scenarios taking place? Most likely not, as they sound incredibly ridiculous. But imagine, if you will, that these scenarios do occur. What will the outcome be for these patients? The newly diagnosed diabetic patient will go home, unprepared to take care of his disease. Since he wasn't told about his diagnosis, he will continue to eat whatever he chooses, sending his blood sugar through the roof. Because he wasn't told how to check his blood sugar or why that is important, the patient doesn't know when to give himself insulin. In addition, even if he did know when to give himself insulin, he wasn't instructed how to do it. How much should he draw up? How does he even draw up the insulin? Without any of this knowledge, the patient will likely suffer complications related to an elevated blood glucose level. The patient will likely need to be seen in the emergency department and subsequently be admitted to the ICU.

What about the new parents with the premature twins? How will these infants eat once they're home if their parents have not received instruction on how to gavage-feed them? All newborns need adequate caloric intake, but this is especially important for preemies. And what about the apnea monitors? If the twins are on apnea monitors, it's likely that they are at risk for disruptions in breathing or heart rate. The parents weren't instructed on how to respond to the alarms, assuming the parents somehow understand how to operate the monitors to begin with. Essentially, the infants' lives are at risk.

The 35-year-old patient who's about to undergo a hysterectomy has no idea why she needs surgery, let alone which organ is being removed. She's never had children, so the implications for a hysterectomy for her are quite significant. Is a hysterectomy even needed, or were there other treatment options?

All of these scenarios demonstrate how patient education is *essential* to the daily operations of any patient care environment. Would any of the aforementioned scenarios be considered "nice to have"? Would any hospital administrator or senior leader deem them "nice to have"? Most likely not, and if they did, I would argue that they do not belong in healthcare. But when budget cuts

 Effectively Managing Patient Education

and other issues arise that threaten the viability of patient education and the services the department delivers, the patient education manager must advocate and demonstrate how these services are indeed *crucial*.

Other challenges relate to resource allocation. Patient education, when buried within the larger centralized education department, also risks being diluted by a larger staff development function that can give a distorted picture of the amount of support available. For example, a centralized education department could have a total of 19 FTEs, only one of whom is devoted exclusively to supporting patient education. This can give the impression that there is a very well-staffed, centralized education department that meets all education needs for the hospital, but in reality, patient education is sorely understaffed.

The existence of these challenges leaves the patient education manager with the burden of ensuring organizational support to meet outcomes that ultimately equate to patient safety and care quality. In this chapter, we will discuss strategies to address these barriers and to garner the attention and support of senior leaders.

Gaining Visibility

You can have brilliant ideas, but if you can't communicate them, your ideas won't get you anywhere.

—*Lee Iacocca*

If managing patient education is a new role (as it often is) for both you and your organization, it can be especially challenging to gain visibility; yet doing so is critical to the success of any patient education initiative, especially one that requires change and subsequent mobilization of a large group of individuals to achieve desired outcomes. The most effective way to gain visibility is to get noticed in your organization while simultaneously gaining credibility. To accomplish this requires a targeted, proactive approach that relies heavily on communication strategies—particularly, communicating the message that patient education is an essential part of healthcare and affects key success measures that senior leaders care about, such as patient satisfaction, patient safety, and alignment with organizational strategic goals.

Senior leaders care about these measures because these are the factors that keep their business alive and competitive. No hospital administrator wants to run a hospital that has a poor patient safety record and low patient satisfaction scores. As healthcare becomes increasingly competitive, patients often "shop around" for healthcare systems that are safe and consumer-driven. Strategic goals are additional ways in which hospitals can advance major initiatives and grow as a business. Senior leaders care about initiatives that help further those goals.

Getting your message across effectively to senior leaders is a skill you must learn early. Through my experience communicating with senior leaders, I've walked away with three essential insights. I've learned to:

- **Speak their language.** Senior leaders generally think in more global terms as the issue relates to the organization, rather than at the unit or department level. If you're trying to persuade a senior leader that additional funding is necessary for patient education, you should demonstrate how this additional support will result in patient education materials getting into the hands of patients more quickly, rather than focusing on relieving your workload—even if that is a natural (and intended) consequence of the additional support.

- **Show data.** Not everyone is data-driven, but generally, senior leaders appreciate seeing how you are arriving at your conclusions. You can bolster your cause by demonstrating the issue with data. For example, when attempting to gain additional funding to pay for translation services for patient education materials, demonstrating the percentage of the population in your hospital's market area that is Spanish-speaking, as well as your admission rates and future trends regarding population growth, will solidify the need and will demonstrate real cause.

- **Wrap it up in a neat package.** It may be tempting to write a lengthy report outlining why you believe a certain change needs to occur, or to come prepared to a meeting with all the possible reasons why leadership needs to accept your proposal; after all, the more information the better, right? Not necessarily. Senior leaders have very limited time to focus on one particular issue. Given the nature of their role, their span of control is often large and they hear a wealth of information daily. Although being knowledgeable in the content is prudent so that you can field questions or take a deeper dive if desired by your audience, an effective way to package up your communication is through the SBAR technique.[1]

Using SBAR (and CRM) as communication tools

Situation background assessment recommendation (SBAR) is a framework for communication that assists you in packaging up your message to communicate the essentials, and allows both the messenger and the receiver to focus on the concrete details without the added burden of having to sort through rhetoric. SBAR was originally developed by Michael Leonard, MD, physician leader for patient safety, along with colleagues Doug Bonacum and Suzanne Graham at Kaiser Permanente of Colorado, in response to the 1999 Institute of Medicine (IOM) report *To Err Is Human: Building a Safer Health System*.[2] SBAR is now being widely used in the healthcare setting, particularly in nurse–physician communication, as a patient safety initiative to alleviate the errors in healthcare that often occur with miscommunication. However, SBAR has its roots in the aviation industry and NASA, where crew resource management (CRM) was developed.[3] CRM was designed in response to the aviation disasters of the 1970s and 1980s to focus on communication and decision-making within a team. (see book excerpt following this section).

Despite SBAR being tailored primarily for nurse–physician communication at the bedside, it's an extremely effective tool for organizing any type of critical communication.

Here is an example of how you would use SBAR in speaking to a senior leader:

S (Situation): Patient education materials currently exist in a decentralized environment. In terms of development, no standards exist for patient education materials in the form of content, branding, or review. An analysis of current materials revealed that our patient education print materials are at too high a reading level for patients to understand.

B (Background): With a decentralized approach, units, departments, and other entities across the enterprise manage patient education on their own, by purchasing, obtaining, or developing unique materials. Patient education needs assessments are conducted at the unit/department level and not at the system level. This leaves room for duplication and redundancy in efforts.

A (Assessment): An enterprisewide audit revealed that we have 11,967 individual patient education documents, with about 80% authored internally. Eighty-five percent of the documents were written at higher than an eighth-grade level. More than 50% of the documents did not contain the organization's logo or branding. Print quality was lacking. A decentralized approach puts our patients at risk because:

- Information varies across units, departments, and entities. Patients are confused about which information is correct.

- Standards for written information cannot be enforced, resulting in information being conveyed at too high a level.

A decentralized approach puts the organization at risk because:

- The community looks to our organization for quality health information that is consistent and at the cutting edge
- Lack of good print quality or a logo does not present a good image to the community

R (Recommendation): Centralize all patient education print material, which allows for:

- Online access across the organization via an online catalog
- Paperless archival, storage, and management of print collateral
- Assurance that patient education standards are met and the organizational image is preserved
- Less duplication and redundancy in effort
- Consistency of clinical information

With the SBAR technique, leaders can quickly understand the issue you are presenting before them and what action you recommend that the organization take. From there, details such as developing the work plan around the action you recommend can be discussed at another meeting or with another group.

In essence, the single largest factor in obtaining organization support is getting your message across effectively. The rest of this chapter will discuss specific ways to leverage varying communication techniques.

The following text is from the HCPro book, *SBAR Basics: A Resource Guide for Healthcare Managers*

The Role of Senior Leadership

Implementing SBAR takes an organizational commitment—it must become part of every clinical department's operations if it is to succeed. As you might expect, hospitalwide implementation will require significant organizational energy and much staff education. Effective implementation must be well-planned in order to succeed, and it will take considerable thought and time. Senior leadership must set the expectation and lead the organization in this new endeavor.

A good place to start might be to locate a hospital similar to yours that has developed an SBAR program and find out roughly how much time, effort, and cost were involved in its implementation.

Building Your SBAR Team

SBAR cannot be implemented in isolation if the organization expects to use it for interdepartmental or interdisciplinary communication. Therefore, it is important to build a solid team first. This SBAR planning team should include:

- The organization's chief nursing officer

- The chief medical officer

- C-suite executives who oversee clinical departments such as radiology, surgery, and emergency

- Medical directors

- Resident program directors

Bear in mind that SBAR won't be an instant success. Even with solid, widespread support, it will take commitment and persistence to bring SBAR into a hospital and make it work. If you encounter resistance from leaders, keep trying. If you can find a champion in the C-suite, enlist his or her help in spreading the word. Unfortunately, it might take a serious incident, publicized error, or undesirable outcome for some people in management to understand that better communication is essential. Often, structured, organized, assertive communication is a foreign concept to most hospital staff members. Therefore, it will take time and practice for SBAR to become part of everyday communication—but it can be done.

For example, Kaiser Permanente in Oakland, CA, has successfully embedded SBAR in its organization by using SBAR in every communication, from executive memos to clinical handoffs. This strategy has helped solidify SBAR into the culture of the organization.[1]

In addition to recruiting leadership, recruit support from other departments, including physicians and nurses from every unit, pharmacy, and other areas. These groups have different priorities, so you must make the case for SBAR using different strategies. These different approaches are discussed below in relation to the barriers you may face when trying to build support among different groups of caregivers.

Barriers to Implementation and Practical Ways to Overcome Them

Consider these six barriers when promoting implementation of any new process:

- Lack of awareness

- Lack of self-efficacy

- Inertia of previous practice

- Lack of familiarity

- Lack of agreement

- Lack of outcome expectancy[2]

In addition, a common barrier to the use of SBAR in healthcare organizations is a hierarchical environment (whether real or perceived) in which nurses are fearful of asserting themselves to physicians, residents are fearful of asserting themselves to their attending physicians, and ancillary staff members are fearful of asserting themselves to nursing staff members.

Address each of these potential barriers before implementing the new strategy.

Creating Awareness and Self-Efficacy

The first step in the change process is to create awareness of the communication problem. Clinicians are often unaware of the magnitude of the effect that their everyday practices can have on their patients. Although many staff members can articulate the need for improved communication, most have not been involved in a sentinel event.

Effectively Managing Patient Education

In addition, when provided with information about sentinel events or other evidence indicating that handoff communication is important, staff members tend to believe that those types of events happen to others, at other institutions. After all, it's much easier to say, "It can't happen here, and it can't happen to me," than it is to commit to making changes for the better.

Heightening awareness of communication problems is only part of the challenge, however. Developing self-efficacy—an understanding that "it can happen here, but there are things that I can do to prevent it"—is another. A review of the facility's trends related to untoward events and poor communication, as well as the use of facility-specific case scenarios, can help create the impetus for change.

If you can't find a scenario from within the organization, use a scenario that comes from a similar environment with which staff members can identify. The scenario must be believable to staff members so that they can identify with it. Staff members need to be able to see the scenario happening within their facility.

Conquering Inertia

How many times have you heard, "But this is how we've *always* done it"? Inertia can be a big obstacle to change of any kind, and, unfortunately, it's one of the most common that you'll encounter. How do you deal with staff members who can't or won't change to accommodate SBAR? You'll need a variety of approaches and incentives.

If your leadership makes it clear that SBAR is an expectation, not a choice, your initiative has a better chance of succeeding. Making it a point to show that upper management is committed to SBAR might convince reluctant caregivers to cooperate.

You'll also have an easier time overcoming inertia if you can convince staff members that using SBAR will improve patient safety and reduce communication breakdowns. Identifying and communicating the need for change for each group that will use the SBAR model is important to achieve buy-in. You may need to use different scenarios for the various stakeholders, because diverse groups will have different needs.

For nurses, the model must allow them to serve successfully as advocates for patient care. Show nurses that SBAR allows them to clearly articulate and request the interventions that their patients need.

Likewise, because physicians are trained to solve problems, they must understand how SBAR will enable them to do so more efficiently. For a physician to take appropriate action, the problem must be identified clearly during the conversation. In my role as director of clinical quality and patient safety, I have had physicians report that they frequently receive calls from nurses and are unable to decipher what the nurse is truly requesting. They also report that when they do not know the nurse personally, it is difficult to determine the request's level of urgency. SBAR provides a consistent approach to the phone calls physicians receive from nursing staff.

Administrators want to avoid the negative publicity and malpractice suits associated with unexpected outcomes, sentinel events, and near misses. If you can identify how the SBAR model for communication will assist in this endeavor, administrators will be more likely to embrace SBAR and advocate for the change. Translating untoward outcomes into dollars spent is another powerful tool that captures senior leadership's attention.

Creating Familiarity and Agreement

Winning organizations start with small pilot tests (e.g., using SBAR for shift change on one nursing unit). Alternatively, picking a handoff between two departments, such as a postoperative care unit and an ICU, can be used for the first rollout.

Finding a few staff members who will champion SBAR is important at the pilot stage. Engage these staff members and recruit them for your pilot team. These staff members will use the tool first and experience the pitfalls as well as the successes, so it is important to recruit people that are enthusiastic about the model and are willing to put effort into making the project work.

One way to find these staff members is to pitch the SBAR solution to a group that has identified handoff communication as an issue. This may occur after a particular event in your organization. If you have trouble identifying such an event, check with your risk manager, who may be able to provide examples of times when more effective communication could have improved a patient's outcome. If the risk manager does not have such an example, ask staff members whether they have ever received incorrect information or were not given enough information about a patient. Let them share this experience. Then watch the group's reaction to your possible solution (SBAR) as you share the scenario you decide to use for an example. Look for potential early adopters.

Once some enthusiasm for trying the SBAR model has been generated, ask whether there are any departments that would like to serve as a pilot. Market your solution first to management staff members, and recruit the units or departments that will be used for the pilot. Next, take the idea to the

Effectively Managing Patient Education

staff members who work in those areas, present the idea to them, and solicit volunteers. Now you have your pilot areas and a team of volunteers engaged!

Another technique is to use SBAR as part of a larger change. For example, when Via Christi Regional Medical Center in Wichita, KS, was starting a rapid response team (RRT), they decided to use the SBAR model to communicate.

The team incorporated education on SBAR communication and the criteria for calling the RRT and included both in the documentation for the RRT. Because the RRT was a completely new concept, this technique allowed staff members to experience using SBAR communication without changing any previous practices.

In any scenario, a small pilot test provides a "laboratory" for a group of committed individuals to try out small changes and learn more about what works in one environment before rolling the model out to an entire organization. The familiar plan-do-study-act (PDSA) model for improvement,[3] which advocates this methodology, has been used by numerous hospitals, including OSF St. Joseph Medical Center in Bloomington, IL,[4] and Bronson Methodist Hospital in Kalamazoo, MI,[5] to implement the SBAR methodology.

References

1. Pillow, M., and V. Smith, eds. 2006. "Using the SBAR Technique." *Improving Handoff Communication* 6 (August): 9–15. Joint Commission on Accreditation of Healthcare Organizations. Oakbrook Terrace, IL.

2. Feldstein, A., and R. Glasgow. 2008. "A Practical, Robust Implementation and Sustainability Model (PRISM) for Integrating Research Findings into Practice." *The Joint Commission Journal on Quality and Patient Safety* 34 (April): 228–243.

3. Langley G., et al. 1996. *The Improvement Guide: A Practical Approach to Enhancing Organizational Performance.* San Francisco: Jossey-Bass.

4. Haig, K.M. 2006. "SBAR: A Shared Mental Model for Improving Communication Between Clinicians." *The Joint Commission Journal on Quality and Patient Safety* 32 (March): 167–175.

The following text is from the HCPro book, *Crew Resource Management: The Flight Plan for Lasting Change in Patient Safety*

Arm Your Team with CRM Skills

Your team won't be complete until it functions with the proper CRM skills. Encourage your team members to keep an open mind when learning the new skills and to practice them for success.

Situational awareness skills—what are they and how do they apply to healthcare?

Situational awareness (SA) is a common aviation term that refers to the ability to make and maintain an accurate assessment of the "big picture" view of what is happening and to predict accurately what might happen based on what is seen at this moment. Pilots are often heard describing difficult emergency situations in terms of how much or how little SA they had at the moment. After a simulator session in which a crew has had to handle both an engine on fire and a hydraulic system failure, you might hear the captain say, "So much was going on that I had low SA and didn't realize we were so close to the mountains."

Because high SA is so important for flight safety, crews spend many hours training to detect warning signs that their SA is low and at risk. Being able to predict results based on current events is critical to avoiding adverse outcomes. The concept of training to recognize warning signs comes from a study of the root causes of multiple air carrier accidents. In the retrospective study, researchers analyzed scores of accidents and asked two questions:

1. Were warning signs present in the events that led up to the accident?

2. If the crew had been trained to recognize the warning signs, could they have detected them in time to avert the unwanted outcome?

Researchers realized that most aviation accidents are preceded by known and detectable warning signs. In each airline accident reviewed in the study, there were no fewer than four indicators or warning signs per accident, and in most of the accidents, seven key indicators were present. Since this landmark study, pilots and crews in both military and commercial aviation have been trained to recognize these warning signs and equipped with actions to take when a warning sign, or red flag, is detected.

Teach your team how to detect and respond to warning signs or red flags

Here is the core list of red flags that should be included in a training program and customized to each organization or specialty:

- **Conflicting input:** Two or more sources of information disagree. Information may come from team members, equipment, charts, etc. For example, air traffic control (ATC) alerts the flight crew that they are 15 miles from their destination airport. However, the onboard navigation equipment indicates that they are only 8 miles from the airport. If this information is not reconciled, the flight may land at the wrong airport—a decided safety risk. In a healthcare example, there have been no alarms from the pulse oximeter, but the patient's blood is very dark due to hypoxia.

- **Preoccupation:** Fixation or intense focus on one task or problem to the exclusion of other potential dangers. Fixation or preoccupation may cause you to ignore other important priorities, such as flying the airplane, fighting a fire, or responding to an important call. Preoccupation has contributed to many aviation accidents, including a well-known tragedy—Eastern Airlines Flight 401—when a jumbo jet slowly descended until it crashed in the Florida Everglades. The pilots were preoccupied with a faulty warning indicator. Caught up in fiddling with a burned-out lightbulb in the landing gear indicator, they were oblivious to the fact that the airplane was slowly descending toward certain death. In healthcare, fixation might lead an anesthesiologist to be preoccupied with placing an endotracheal tube while ignoring the pulse oximeter and the patient's dangerously low oxygen levels.

- **Not communicating:** Team members do not ask for or offer input to one another. Additionally, one team member may ask a question, but receive no reply. Note that "not communicating" does not always mean there is no talking among the team. Often, there is talking, but no real communication. For example, comments may not be acknowledged or questions may go unanswered.

- **Confusion:** A situation characterized by doubt as to what is really happening. Two behaviors are associated with this red flag—unanswered questions from one team member to another, and thinking, "This is stupid," "This doesn't make sense," or "Why is it/the patient doing this?"

- **Violating regulations or standard operating procedure:** A team member or the whole team exceeds established limits or does not follow normal procedures, and no one mentions or questions the intended course of action.

- **Failure to set/meet targets:** Examples are the easiest way to describe this red flag. Here's an aviation example: The flight plan for a flight from Memphis, TN, to Los Angeles will clearly indicate the amount of fuel required to fly that distance. At each checkpoint along the route of flight, the flight plan indicates how much fuel should be remaining in the tanks to complete the flight safely to destination. Let's say the flight plan indicates 24,000 lbs of fuel should be in the tanks as the airplane flies over Oklahoma City, but there are only 21,000 lbs of fuel in the tanks. This is a warning sign: The airplane needs 24,000 lbs of fuel to complete the flight, but only has 21,000 lbs—the target has not been met.

In healthcare, let's say that a certain surgical procedure normally requires about an hour and a half to complete. But one hour into the procedure, only one-quarter of the necessary steps have been accomplished. This might be a red flag. The normal time target is not being met, and that may be indicative of a more serious condition, which should alert the team to watch for other warning signs of a potential adverse outcome.

- **Not addressing discrepancies:** Unresolved confusion, doubts, concerns, and unmet targets that are not brought to the attention of the team. There is almost universal agreement in healthcare organizations that in most sentinel events and patient-harming incidents, at least one member of the team was aware that something was amiss yet failed to address the issue with other members of the team.

The presence of a red flag does not guarantee an adverse outcome or incident. Detecting one red flag should merely alert team members to watch for the presence of additional red flags. As previously noted in the study, every aircraft accident had at least four red flags. Detecting more than one red flag in a given situation should bring the team to a heightened level of concern and awareness.

Knowing what action to take when red flags are detected is as important as recognizing them in the first place. The actions to take can be described by the statement, "See it, say it, and fix it." By "see it," we mean that team members must be trained to detect red flags and be alert for their presence. "Say it" represents the act of speaking up about what is seen and alerting others on the team to the red flag. "Fix it" means taking the action needed at that moment to stop the chain of events from causing patient harm. Often, no action is needed other than to verbally note the red flag. At other times, the discrepancy causing the red flag must be fixed by specific action appropriate for the situation.

How Should Team Skills Be Taught to Healthcare Professionals?

The answer to this question lies in the full understanding that these are "skills" or learned behaviors and actions that healthcare providers take. Aviation training designers refer to CRM as "things people do." Therefore, the skills-based seminars should incorporate these four requirements for adult learning:

- **Motivation:** Each skill module should clearly answer these questions: Why is this important to me? What is the payoff for the physician or staff member who uses this skill? How will incorporating this skill set help staff members improve their practice, provide better care for their patients, and keep their patients safer?

- **Practice:** New skills take practice. The curriculum design must allow the participants to use each of the skills they are learning or improving. This requires an instructional plan that includes case studies and other experiential activities that require participants to speak and act using the desired behaviors.

- **Reinforcement (or feedback):** CRM course facilitators must be experts at providing feedback to the participants on the use of the skills during the learning activities. Expert facilitators can discriminate among varying levels of teamwork performance and are adept at coaching participants to meet the desired skill level. Medical personnel are not typically trained to provide this level of facilitation and coaching skill. Facilitators must be chosen carefully and extensively trained. Quick train-the-trainer courses or brief periods with a consultant are not usually successful and should be viewed with caution.

- **Transfer:** What is learned in the classroom must be transferable to the hospital or clinic environment. The greatest learning transfer occurs when the fidelity of what happens in the classroom is closely aligned to the real world. In other words, the realism and accuracy of the learning activities become important to real and lasting skill improvement. Organizations choosing to work with consultants to implement CRM programs must ensure that the consultants have a depth of experience with healthcare that enables them to create learning activities with the highest fidelity to the real world of medicine.

Communication campaigns

One of the more effective communication strategies is an internal communication campaign. A communication campaign's purpose is to expose weaknesses within the organization, under the auspices of patient safety, and to offer solutions in a manner that is informational, as opposed to dogmatic. Coming across as too authoritarian, especially in a new role, can be seen as overstepping your authority, and your message may be disregarded.

A communication campaign needs to touch on safety issues, financial effect, and the current state of the organization. The results of your literature search and environmental assessment of your organization will guide what should be communicated. For example, your organizational assessment may reveal that patient education materials are consistently written at a tenth-grade level or higher. Therefore, an assumption could be made that the organization is lacking awareness of health literacy and the importance of communicating in ways that patients can understand and act on. As a result of this finding, the basics of health literacy would be a suitable topic to cover in a communication campaign.

Health literacy is an emerging area of study and research that is not yet well understood by healthcare organizations and providers, yet it has an enormous effect on patients and their families, staff members, and healthcare expenditures. (Chapter 4 provides more detailed information regarding health literacy.) As the patient education manager, here is an opportunity to not only gain visibility, but also introduce a very important topic and link it to things that senior leaders care about, such as patient safety, patient satisfaction, and budget implications.

Lifespan of a communication campaign

A communication campaign might begin in a nonconfrontational and unassuming way, through e-mail "teasers." Teasers present information in such a fashion as to spur interest to the point that the audience will want additional, in-depth information. Figure 2.1 is an example of an e-mail teaser.

| FIGURE 2.1 | E-mail teaser example |

To: All Clinical Leadership

From: Patient Education Manager

Re: Is This Your Patient?

"A baby was brought to the clinic with diarrhea. I treated the baby and told the mother to 'push fluids' with the baby. That was about 8 a.m. The mother brought the baby home, and at noon the baby was dead. The mother had literally pushed fluids by tipping the baby's bottle upside down and forcing the fluid when the baby's responses began to slow down. The baby suffocated." (Doak, et al., 1996)

Is this your patient?

Not if you're aware that as many as 27 million Americans, 1 out of 5, are estimated to be functionally illiterate.

Not if you're aware that the average reading level of most Americans is below eighth grade.

Not if you're aware that poor readers interpret directions literally, without accounting for new situations/contexts.

Chances are high that the patients you see on a regular basis suffer from low health literacy. Be a health literacy champion and use simpler communication with your patients.

Attached is an example of Words to Watch in Patient Education—concept words to help you communicate with patients and their families.

As always, if you have questions or concerns, please don't hesitate to contact me.

Thank you, and happy educating!!

Reference: Doak, C., Doak, L., and Root, J. *Teaching Patients with Low Literacy Skills* (New York: Lippincott, 1996).

The role of early adopters

Those who are looking for additional information are generally "early adopters"; these individuals are willing to cautiously try out new ideas, and they are important to identify because they can assist in becoming agents of change, allowing you to then build a slow, steady momentum of change. Several theories about change exist, but one commonly held belief is the Rogers Model for the Adoption and Diffusion of Innovations.[4] This model classifies adopters of change into various categories, reminding us that the momentum of change is a process.

Early adopters account for roughly 13.5% of your audience, and they are individuals who are often viewed as opinion leaders. The "early majority" represents approximately 34% of the audience, and accepts change much more quickly than the average person. The "late majority" generally comprises skeptics who will acquiesce to new ideas or patterns only after the majority has already done so. This group represents 34% of your audience. Finally, the remaining 16% or so are "laggards," and these are the people who are often highly critical of new ways and ideas and tend to accept them only when they become "tradition."

Keeping this model in mind is useful when trying to impart large-scale change quickly and en masse. This is why identifying early adopters and investing in their energy will make the transition to change occur much more smoothly. Your early adopters are your greatest asset in building momentum at the grassroots level. Simply put, if you were the single voice for patient education, it would be extremely challenging for you to single-handedly get your message across to the entire organization. The early adopters can take your message and convey the need for, and importance of, your initiative to staff members whom you can't reach well, such as second- and third-shift staff members, as well as other nonclinical staff members who, unbeknownst to you, are involved in communicating/educating patients.

The lifespan of the communication campaign then continues to leadership presentations (including one-on-one meetings as needed) and ends by reaching out directly to clinical/bedside staff members. Presenting to these two groups requires you to be dynamic in your approach and adjust your communication technique accordingly.

Presenting to leadership

Presenting for the first time to a leadership group can be intimidating, but with a bit of preparation, your presentation should go smoothly. First, dress to impress. If you are not a titled leader (yet), it's important that you nevertheless dress like one, especially when standing in front of a

Effectively Managing Patient Education

group of leaders. Your audience, right or wrong, will make assumptions about your authority and credibility based on your clothes. Second, take time to plan your presentation. Even if you are intimately familiar with the topic and feel like you could speak forever, *don't*. Chances are you were graciously given a certain amount of time on the agenda to present, and you should stick to that time frame. Similar to how you prepare a patient education document, determine the main things you want your audience to walk away knowing, and construct your presentation with that in mind. Finally, make sure you end your presentation with what you are specifically asking leadership to do (an action item) as a result of the information you presented to them. For example, whether are you asking for their support or for them to specifically *do* something (such as be a member of a committee), be sure this is very clear.

An example of a PowerPoint presentation to leadership can be found on the CD-ROM included with this book; this particular presentation was made in less than 10 minutes as part of an effort to keep hospital leaders up-to-date with patient education efforts and concluded with interest from leaders in being part of a new systemwide patient education committee.

It's critical to target the vice presidents of nursing or patient care, medical chiefs, and other clinical managers in your leadership presentations and e-mail teasers; these influential individuals govern the heart and soul of the hospital, which is direct patient care. Their staff members touch patients every day, and as such, they provide patient education. Although ultimately your messages need to reach those groups, to get to them requires gaining the support of their vice president. In addition, having the support of such a person can help you remove barriers to initiating the change you wish to see.

Reaching out to the clinical staff

It's always a challenge to reach out to the clinical staff. As patient education managers, we generally work set hours during the day shift and, with few exceptions, rarely leave our offices other than for meetings here and there. Rarely do we have the opportunity to stand in front of the entire nursing work force in a hospital and give a presentation. But there are some ways to get your message out.

First, ask to come to department staff meetings. (This could be that "action item" you asked for support in when you gave your leadership presentation.) Here you have a captive audience and are going directly to staff members in their environment. By using the department staff meeting as your venue, you also give the impression that leadership finds the information worthwhile, since they are devoting meeting time to your topic. Second, having key points available for staff members to look at on their own is an effective way to convey information, without coming across as mandatory reading.

An effective method that worked in my organization was developing an attractive poster that was placed in the cafeteria, with "tear-off" sheets so that staff members could easily take a handout that listed key points. The tear-off sheets were very well received. Figures 2.2 and 2.3 are examples of tear-off sheets.

FIGURE 2.2   **Health literacy tear-off sheet example**

Low Health Literacy

Making Sure Your Patients "Get It"

What is health literacy?

Health literacy is the ability to read, understand, and act on health information. But nearly half of all Americans (90 million) have difficulty understanding health information, such as discharge instructions, patient education handouts, and medication labels. Most adults cannot read above an eighth-grade level.

Who has low health literacy?

Studies show that on average, adults in the United States read three to five levels below their years of education.

Also:

- 75% of Americans with a chronic disease have limited literacy
- 66% of adult Americans age 60 or older have marginal literacy skills
- 50% of welfare recipients read below a fifth-grade level
- 50% of Hispanic-Americans have reading problems
- 40% of African-Americans have reading problems

Red flags:

- Eyes wander over the page
- Shows lack of interest in reading materials
- Shows frustration or impatience with reading materials
- Says "I forgot my glasses" or "my eyes are tired"
- Looks at the pills instead of at the pill bottle label

How to help your patients:

Make them comfortable. "Many people have trouble with these materials. How can I help?"
Assess. "What do you like to read?" or "How happy are you with the way you read?"
Offer materials that are written at no higher than a sixth-grade level.

FIGURE 2.3 Education tips

PATIENT EDUCATION TIPS

Medications

Using Education to Ensure Safe Practices

Every patient who is admitted to our facilities is started on at least *one new medication*, in addition to the medications he or she was already on at home. The average number of medications a patient can be on is estimated to be about 16.

What do patients need to know?

BEFORE administering medications to patients, they should be told:

- The name of their medication
- What the medication is for
- Frequent side effects
- Any contraindications or special considerations with the medication

To help make learning easier for your patients:

- **Provide written drug information** *in addition* to your verbal instruction. Also remember that the best source of accurate and complete drug information is the pharmacist!
- **Include family members and/or caregivers** during your medication teaching, so they can provide reminders and help remember information.
- **Do not wait until discharge** to begin educating the patient about his or her medications.
- **Clearly explain the directions,** including obvious information. For example, some teens have spread contraceptive jelly on their toast and have eaten it, thinking it would provide birth control.
- **Always utilize the teach-back method** to fully assess patient understanding.
- **Identify patients at risk for noncompliance;** consider a homecare referral or partner with the pharmacy to offer a different dosing schedule or regime that may eliminate errors or confusion at home.
- **Document** your assessment and teaching! This allows all disciplines to follow up as appropriate and plan care accordingly.

Reference: Institute for Safe Medication Practices, 2007

Dense fog advisory: Visibility challenges, and tactics to overcome them

As fog gets thicker, it gets increasingly difficult to see and navigate without serious blunders. The same is true for a lack of clarity in a communication campaign. Some trouble spots can include:

- Over- or underexerting your authority

- Inadvertently skipping the chain of command

- Simply not being fully aware of the hospital or healthcare system's political landscape

Such are the challenges to gaining visibility. For example, getting on the leadership agenda is one thing; *staying* on it is another. When leaders aren't fully aware of the importance of your message (as we discussed in the preceding example regarding health literacy), you risk being bumped off the agenda for other important topics to be discussed or presented. Here is where the patient education manager needs to appeal to his or her reporting director or vice president to wield influence to get back on the agenda. And although this may work for a period of time, sooner or later the patient education manager will need to wield his or her own influence. Achieving this level of influence can be challenging.

To address this challenge, the person responsible for managing patient education at the system level needs to be a titled leader, for the following reasons:

- It levels the playing field for the patient education manager with other clinical leadership, and therefore allows a certain amount of authority and influence to be exerted without as much fear of a political misstep

- It allows for greater autonomy and less reliance on the reporting director or vice president to get things done or solve problems

- It strengthens the perceived importance of the patient education function across the organization, allowing for ease in gaining and maintaining support

- It allows greater access to information such as strategic goal planning and organizational updates, which are crucial for planning for patient education

If the patient education role is not a titled leadership position, you still can accomplish the goals in the preceding list, but it will likely happen at a much slower pace and with several hurdles along the way.

Finally, the most valuable asset any new patient education manager should have is a mentor. Ideally, a mentor is someone within the organization who is at a senior leadership level and who can offer guidance in navigating the organization's political landscape, provide valuable feedback, and give insightful coaching. You can gain a mentor at the senior leadership level by being visible while gaining credibility, and utilizing the communication campaign mentioned earlier.

Quite honestly, patient education within my organization went from being an ignored and hidden issue to one that is discussed often and is highly visible. This can be attributed to my mentor relationship with one of the more senior-level executives in the organization. The idea of my bringing health literacy awareness to the organization captured her attention, originally through communication campaigns I had launched. When I started in my role, I sent these communication campaign e-mails to every e-mail leadership distribution list I could find: nursing directors, management, clinical leadership, and so on. This is how I found my mentor. I wasn't even sure *who* was on those e-mail lists, but I figured that if they were on the lists, they needed to know what I was communicating. In fact, many people in my organization say they first heard my name from people who were talking about the latest e-mail I had sent regarding health literacy.

My mentor and I have a great relationship, and we seem to have the same approach to issues, although I admit to sometimes feeling uncertain about how to utilize her support. I value the time she spends to mentor me (30 minutes every other month) and that she takes interest in my professional growth, yet simultaneously, I sometimes feel like I am wasting her time. Our agenda when we meet is completely open-ended and set by me—whatever I would like to discuss or whatever is on my mind. In fact, she often opens the discussion with: "How are things?" or "What is on your mind?" Here is where I initially started filtering what I would say; should I start to complain about how I felt the organization wasn't ready for an expanded and integrated patient education approach, or should I talk about how I thought the last meeting I was in went well? Or both? After a while, I began to talk about both, showing her that both issues were important to me. Each month we meet, our relationship evolves and we get to know each other better.

Although my communication campaign was effective in finding a mentor, other methods of acquiring a mentor simply include asking your reporting director for a recommendation, or asking a senior leader outright. Most leaders welcome the opportunity to mentor others, so take advantage of this highly valuable experience.

 Effectively Managing Patient Education

Ensure ongoing communication with leadership

Even after the initial wave of e-mails and presentations, it's still very important to keep patient education on leaders' minds. The more information these senior leaders have, the more engaged they will be. In my experience, many leaders have operated on the assumption that if they don't hear any updates about a particular topic, the topic "went away" and was a "flavor of the day" rather than a popular initiative, or that the topic was taken care of and no further action or support was needed from them. This is why it's critical to keep communicating with your leaders. Here are some ways to keep administrators aware of patient education strategies:

- Write to them about the strategies in quarterly memos and annual reports. These high-level reports and memos should contain status updates and accomplishments at the system level (see Figure 2.4).

- Share recent literature findings related to patient education.

- Route meeting minutes and patient education newsletters (see Figure 2.5 for an example of such a newsletter; modify the newsletter sample to fit your organization).

- Present at annual leadership meetings.

- Invite them to educational offerings on patient education topics, including continuing medical education classes for the medical staff.

Communication, both verbally and in writing, is a skill that cannot be overemphasized. In addition to gaining exposure and credibility, it's also an essential tool to keep hospital administrators aware of the status of various patient education initiatives.

| FIGURE 2.4 | Memo about patient education initiatives |

Memo

To: Chief Nursing Officers; Chief Integration Officer
From: Patient Education Coordinator
CC: Education Director
Date: July 7, 2008
Re: Quarterly System Patient Education Update

Patient Education Initiatives

The purpose of this memo is to communicate the status of various patient education initiatives as Community Hospital moves toward an aligned, patient-centered approach with patient education. To date, the system has realized the following accomplishments toward this goal:

- The **Patient & Family Education Committee** has been successfully meeting for over one year with growing membership and energy.

- The patient education inventory audit commenced January 2008 as the first step in the work plan toward one aligned patient education catalog. **Total inventory as of June 20, 2008: > 3,500 total patient education pieces. Goal: 1000.**

- Enhanced **patient education flow sheet** in the EMR, allowing ease of documentation and introduction of new Patient Response Scale; pilot phase with diabetes education to go into production July 17, 2008. Championed at the department level by diabetic resource nurses throughout the system.

- Alignment of patient education policies across the system: new **Patient Education Practice Standards** policy set to be implemented, which reduces confusion, drives users to document in only one place, and outlines best practice.

- **Patient & Family Resource Center** at expanded services to include open access, effective Monday July 2. Traffic volumes have doubled from average of 1 patron/hour to 2 patrons/hour.

 Effectively Managing Patient Education

FIGURE 2.5	Sample patient education newsletter

Patient Education Matters

Fall 2008	Volume 1, Number 2

In This Issue

- **Health Literacy: What You Can Do About It**
- **Introducing . . . the Patient Education Team!**
- **Patient Education Mission and Vision Statement**
- **Legal Issues: Nurse Sued for Talking Down to Patient**

Fall Is in the Air!

It's hard to believe it's already time for the second issue of *Patient Education Update*, now called *Patient Education Matters*! In the short amount of time since we began this newsletter, we have seen a lot of activity regarding patient education at _(insert facility here)_. Be sure to read this newsletter to keep current on all that is happening.

Of particular importance is the month of October, as this is when we recognize health literacy, often called the *silent epidemic*. Low health literacy impacts nearly 90 million Americans. ***More people are affected by low health literacy than by diabetes, heart disease, or cancer.***

This issue focuses on some ways to help combat this huge health problem. Remember that you can't tell someone can't read just by looking at him or her!

Health Literacy: What You Can Do About It

I've found that one of the more frustrating issues regarding low health literacy is how hidden the problem is. It doesn't carry outward signs, such as an abnormal lab value or assessment finding, and no one group or population is most at risk. It's almost completely silent. In fact, in one study, physicians could identify only **20%** of their patients who were at the lowest literacy level (third grade). Only 20%! The rest of their patients with low literacy went undetected. And because of the social stigma and shame attached to not being able to read well, patients will often do their best to hide their limitation. In fact, 67% never told their own spouses and 85% never told their coworkers they couldn't read well. They most certainly won't tell you, either.

Why Worry About It?

Health literacy is one of *the* strongest predictors of health status—more than age, income, employment status, race, ethnicity, or education level. When patients can't read or understand their health information, they will most likely end up back in the hospital, be admitted to the ICU, or make medication errors. As a result, they cost the healthcare system up to **$58 billion per year.**

FIGURE 2.5 Sample patient education newsletter (cont.)

What Should You Do About It?

First, recognize that this is a huge health problem, and realize that **one out of every five patients you will see today** will not be able to read the health information, discharge instructions, medication labels, or handouts you give to him or her. Second, be on the lookout for the following "red flags" that may indicate a person is having trouble reading:

· Eyes appear to wander over a page

· Shows lack of interest in or frustration or impatience with written materials

· Takes a long time to fill out forms

· Offers excuses such as "I forgot my glasses" or "My eyes are tired"

· *Looks at* the pills instead of *reading* the label on the pill bottle

Third, offer a **shame-free environment**. Offering a shame-free environment means creating a comfort level for patients who wouldn't otherwise feel comfortable telling you they have trouble reading. This includes offering materials that are written at or less than a sixth-grade level, and talking to patients so that they understand what you're saying without being overwhelmed with terms and medical jargon. Another great way to approach this is to say things such as the following:

"A lot of people have trouble understanding these materials. How can I help you?"

Recognizing health literacy concerns and taking a gentle approach to addressing them can help make the difference between a patient remaining healthy and safe, and a patient becoming frustrated and overwhelmed with health information and being left to figure out what to do on his or her own.

Introducing . . . The Patient Education Team

The month of July marked a first for our facility: formation of the ***Patient & Family Education Team***, the first interdisciplinary, system-level patient education committee. This group is responsible for directing patient education efforts for the organization. The large task of capturing patient education for the entire system and recommending new policies and procedures for how patient education is developed and approved was one of the committee's first concerns, with an anticipated new policy and procedure ready for rollout January 1, 2009. The team is represented by leadership in nursing, pharmacy, radiology, HIM, quality management, and marketing, and meets the first Friday of every month. _____, our patient education coordinator, chairs the team and has a public distribution list in Outlook.

Effectively Managing Patient Education

FIGURE 2.5 Sample patient education newsletter (cont.)

Patient Education Resources

Do you know what patient education resources are available?

- **Cardiology Materials**: a centralized distribution center for cardiovascular materials for both hospitals. For more info, contact Cardiology.
- **Patient Education Videos**: educational videos and programming available for patient viewing.

At the clinics:

The Patient Channel: 12

TIGR On Demand: Channels 91–94

CARE Channel: 8

At the hospitals:

The Patient Channel: 46

TIGR On Demand: Channels 47–50

CARE Channel: 51

Newborn Channel: 52

Newborn Channel Espanola: 53

Patient Education Mission Statement

We support patients, families, and the community in their search for health and well-being by providing quality patient education that is informative and individualized. We believe in empowering patients and their families, and encouraging an active partnership between our healthcare providers and the people they serve.

Vision Statement

Providing an interdisciplinary framework for which patient education can be fully integrated throughout the organization, and the health care continuum.

Legal Issues: Nurse Sued for Talking Down to Patient

Sounds a bit far-fetched, doesn't it? In reality, patients can sue for just about anything. Whether they win is another story.

In 2005, a nurse caring for a patient in her home in Georgia attempted to provide instruction to the patient on how to self-care for her PICC line. The patient felt the instructions and expectations of her were out of line and as such refused to learn the care. The nurse threatened loss of insurance coverage of home health visits, and as a result the patient sued for emotional distress at the fear of losing home care. The case was thrown out after being heard by the Georgia Court of Appeals, but the lesson remains the same: The patient wasn't receptive to the learning methods and materials that were provided to her. The nurse was found to have acted according to policy and procedure and within physician orders, but one task was left undone, and that was patient education. Perhaps a different technique would have worked.

More and more patients are finding fault with the *way* providers communicate as opposed to *what* they are communicating. Keep your communication with your patients friendly, open, and above all, simple. For tips on simple communication, visit **www.askme3.org.**

Created and Distributed by Patient & Family Education Services

Connecting the Dots

Patient education has far-reaching implications on patient safety and satisfaction, staff satisfaction, and organizational goal setting. Patient education intersects with all of these "large dots." As discussed earlier in this chapter, you cannot adhere to patient safety if patients are not educated about their diseases, their conditions, or techniques to stay healthy and out of the hospital. At the same time, patients will not be particularly happy with their hospital experience if they aren't given enough information or education. They often go home unsure about what they need to do to take care of themselves, and as a result they become angry at the healthcare system for not providing them with this information. Subsequently, they may rate that hospital experience poorly.

Another "large dot" item, organizational goal setting, relates to how the organization as a whole will prioritize its resources. Linking patient education activities to those goals and demonstrating how they advance the organization's business plans will help to ensure that resources for patient education are provided.

But in addition to all of that, the bottom line is that ". . . patients and families have the right to be informed; that professional standards describe appropriate patient education; that health care organizations and the law require patient education; and that patients, health care organizations, and society benefit from the process."[5] And although this may be obvious to the patient education manager, it may not be so obvious to leadership, due to other competing priorities or initiatives.

It's our job, therefore, to make those connections and demonstrate how patient education fits into the larger picture for many "large dot" items. Those "large dot" items are patient safety, patient satisfaction, and strategic goals. To connect the dots, the patient education manager must be well-versed in the latest literature findings, be up to date on healthcare trends, and continuously monitor patient satisfaction data.

Patient safety

The issue of patient safety has captured the interest of the public since the IOM's report *To Err Is Human: Building a Safer Health System*,[2] a shocking look into the world of medical errors in hospitals. That report revealed that as many as 98,000 people die each year from medical errors. In response to the report, many professional organizations, clinical research groups, and other government agencies established safety initiatives, goals, and metrics. By 2005, the federal government enacted the Patient Safety and Quality Improvement Act of 2005 (Public Law 109-41), designed to promote a "just" system wherein healthcare professionals can voluntarily report patient safety concerns in an effort to make improvements, without fear of the data being used against them.[6] Prior to this, there were two major barriers to reporting medical errors and/or patient safety events:

- **Fear:** Physicians, nurses, and other staff members were often fearful of litigation or damage to their own professional reputations if medical errors were reported

- **Data isolation:** Patient safety event reports were not collected in a standardized fashion, thus making it difficult to aggregate data and discover trends in the events that might lead to resolution[18]

As a result, the IOM report made the case for the formation of Patient Safety Organizations (PSO), and the Patient Safety and Quality Improvement Act of 2005 allowed that to occur. The purpose of PSOs is to provide privilege and confidentiality so that healthcare organizations and clinicians have a means to report, analyze, and trend patient safety event reports, ultimately allowing for safer delivery of patient care. In fall 2008, information regarding which organizations would become PSOs became available, as did the common formats that spell out how the data provided by hospitals will be collected. For more information about PSOs, visit *www.pso.ahrq.gov/*.

Healthcare organizations have adopted the "culture of safety" movement, which works to ensure that decisions, policies, and procedures are data-driven and transparent, thereby resulting in a learning organization.[7] This culture of safety removes the element of blame and allows healthcare workers to report errors freely, working toward improvements. Imagine a healthcare environment that does not adopt a culture of safety, but rather is fear-based. Patient safety events, such as near misses and other events, would not be reported and instead would go underground. How could anyone learn from an event to prevent it from happening again?

Research has shown that many medical errors in healthcare are not the result of an individual's competence or skill level, but of system failures. Those system failures would not be identified and, subsequently, have no hope of being repaired if the error were not reported and analyzed. Promoting a culture of safety keeps the focus off punitive measures for errors and on keeping patients safe.

The Joint Commission's National Patient Safety Goals directly link patient education's importance to patient safety initiatives. (Refer to Figure 1.4 in Chapter 1 to see which Goals involve patient education.) These Goals specifically identify how patient education is a necessary component in patient safety, such as by educating patients and their families about their medications, anticoagulant therapy (which is a high-risk/high-alert medication), multidrug-resistant organisms, and patient safety practices. Additionally, other studies have demonstrated patient education's importance in keeping patients safe,[8] even without these mandates from an outside organization.

Think back to the scenarios presented earlier in this chapter. Are Joint Commission regulations or National Patient Safety Goals the first things that came to your mind as reasons why patient education should have been provided? Or did you realize that safe, quality patient care was conspicuously absent in those scenarios, because the one item missing from them was patient education? Essentially, safe patient care cannot happen without patient education.

The patient's experience in the acute care setting is one that can reasonably be controlled via staffing numbers, clinician expertise, technologies and treatments available, and policies and procedures. But once patients leave our care, their continued health and safety depends largely on what information and education we arm them and their families with before discharge. If education isn't offered or isn't provided in an understandable manner, or if educational messages are inconsistent across entities or healthcare providers, patients won't know how to take care of themselves at home and will likely suffer a relapse, injure themselves further, or exacerbate their condition, often requiring a readmission or an emergency room visit. In fact, patient safety is a measurement of how effective patient education is prior to discharge, as patient safety tends to increase with effective patient education.[9]

Sitting on the hospital's patient safety committee is an effective way to ensure that patient education is taken into context within patient safety initiatives. Hospital-based patient safety committees are interdisciplinary committees designed to analyze hospital patient safety incidents, in an effort to understand patient safety risks and hopefully mitigate them. They also act to develop policies and procedures related to maintaining a culture of safety within the hospital. As a patient education manager, your role on this committee is:

- To be aware of patient safety events in your facility and to understand how patient education may have played a role.

- To utilize the patient safety committee as a method of support for patient education initiatives that you would like to enact. For example, if you want to reformat the informed consents in your hospital to be more patient-friendly, ask the patient safety committee at large to help implement this.

- To formalize the relationship between patient safety and patient education.

- To increase your visibility in the organization and establish your credibility as a patient education expert with fellow leaders.

Patient satisfaction

Healthcare organizations are continuously monitoring and using patient satisfaction scores as an indicator of success for many initiatives and projects. Patient satisfaction is one way in which an organization can stay competitive in a very volatile healthcare market that is increasingly consumer-driven. Patients are now "shopping" for healthcare, becoming more informed and choosy. Hospitals can't afford to leave their patients dissatisfied. A dissatisfied patient will go somewhere else, taking his or her business and money with him or her. With rising healthcare costs, patients want to be assured that they are getting the best service for their money, and healthcare is increasingly becoming more service-oriented as a result. If a hospital or facility begins to suffer in terms of patient satisfaction, that information is typically posted where potential patients can review and compare the data. And patients will likely steer clear of a hospital that appears to have problems in customer service. Hospital administrators and senior leaders pay close attention to patient satisfaction scores and anything that had a direct effect on them. Hospitals routinely collect and analyze patient satisfaction scores for their own internal interests.

Patient education does have a tremendous effect on patient satisfaction and is a distinct quality indicator.[10] Patient satisfaction can be directly influenced by whether patients receive conflicting information from providers,[11] whether information, particularly perioperative information, is realistic,[12] and whether they are receiving "enough" information postoperatively.[13] Furthermore, patient education has been found to have a significant effect on patients' perceptions of care quality and their overall impression.[14]

The implementation of Hospital Consumer Assessment of Healthcare Providers and Systems (HCAHPS) took patient satisfaction to an entirely different level when it launched in October 2006.[15] This instrument qualitatively measures patients' perceptions of their hospital experience. The survey asks patients 27 questions that fall in one of six domains: communication with physicians, communication with nurses, communication about medications, quality of nursing services, discharge planning, and pain management. In addition, because it is a standardized instrument used nationally and its results are reported publicly, it allows for consumer benchmarking and comparisons. It is the first national, standardized, and publicly reported survey of patients' perspectives.

HCAHPS was developed in partnership with the Centers for Medicare & Medicaid Services and the Agency for Healthcare Research and Quality with the following three goals in mind:

- Produce comparable data on patients' perspectives of care that allows objective and meaningful comparisons between hospitals on topics that consumers determine to be important to them.

- Provide public reporting of the survey results that is designed to create incentives for hospitals to improve quality of care.

- Produce public reporting that will enhance accountability in healthcare by increasing the transparency of the quality of hospital care.[15] The National Quality Forum endorsed the HCAHPS survey instrument in May 2005 and implemented it nationwide in October 2006.[15]

March 28, 2008 was the day the first set of national HCAHPS data became available.[16] An analysis of that report by Jha, Orav, Zheng, and Epstein concluded that overall, hospitals have room for improvement in patients' perception of care. The researchers note that patients' perceptions of their care are of interest because they do "affect the bottom line."[16] This type of data helps consumers choose their care providers and helps hospitals make improvements to retain patients and attract new ones.

Hospitals' HCAHPS results will be posted on the Hospital Compare Web site, found at *www.hospitalcompare.hhs.gov* or from a link on *www.medicare.gov*.[15]

Significant research demonstrates the strong correlation between patient education and overall patient satisfaction. As a patient education manager, receiving and monitoring your organization's patient satisfaction scores and data is necessary to understanding how patient education is or is not playing a role in the scores. How the data is transcribed and communicated across the organization may vary by institution, so you may need to conduct a bit of research and/or ask your reporting director for help in getting access to the data. Generally, the data is reported on a monthly basis. Often the data will be in numeric form, showing how each unit or department is performing overall. But I have found some of the more valuable data to be the patient comments that accompany surveys. In my organization, these comments are compiled into a report by the quality department and are shared across the organization every month. I review them for comments that pertain to patient education and log them to determine whether there are any trends. Depending on what the information yields, I may use it to justify the rationale for an improvement project related to patient education or additional funding to address a problem area.

Organizational goals and strategic initiatives

Strategic goals and initiatives are drivers for how to do your work and to assist in prioritizing activities. They are directives from the highest levels of the organization that determine what the organization will focus on for the next year or two, and they contain specifics on how to attain those goals. Strategic goals are generally systemwide, cascading down to individual departments, which set subgoals to help meet the strategic organizational goals. Any initiative at the department level that can demonstrate alliance with or support of the organizational goals generally will be given preference in dedicated resources. For example, if the organization has a strategic goal to implement patient-/family-centered care across the system, a department goal that supports that strategy might be retooling all patient education handouts to contain patient-centered communication methods. Given its support of the strategic goal, this department goal would be prioritized accordingly.

Since strategic goals are meant to determine the course the overall organization is taking, linking patient education to those goals is a way to help ensure that patient education remains visible and that any initiatives related to patient education are more likely to receive priority, funding, and resources. Communicate the linkage in annual reports on patient education, or in presentations that are shared with senior leaders.

For example, in my organization, I have been advocating for more comprehensive patient and family education services that go beyond providing and maintaining patient education materials. I wrote proposals, gave presentations, and communicated this to my reporting director. Ultimately, achieving this goal involved getting resources in short supply, such as FTEs and budget dollars; thus, it would be difficult to operationalize in isolation. I was able to link this concept of expanding patient and family education services to a large strategic initiative of advancing patient-centered care at our facility. Patient education is an integral component of patient-centered care, so the fit was natural. And recognizing that we need to further explore what that really means, I was also able to add "define patient education needs for the organization" to the strategic work plan. See Figure 2.6 for a sample list of organizational goals and their link to patient education.

FIGURE 2.6	Organizational goals and strategies

Strategic goal	Patient education link
Waste reduction	Centralized, electronic patient education catalog
Staff satisfaction	Enhanced communication of patient/family education services to the staff; increase staff support
Patient-centered care	Patient-centered communication strategies; patient/family resource center
Enhanced community image	Branding of patient education; community education classes

Understanding how patient education fits into the larger landscape of healthcare and the hospital setting is vital to ensuring that programs get the attention and, subsequently, the resources needed to make improvements and grow. Without the support and engagement of senior leadership, patient education is at risk for being underfunded, reprioritized, and potentially eliminated in favor of other competing services and priorities.

A great resource that every patient education manager should have to help him or her effectively persuade others, especially when funding is at risk, is the best-seller about negotiation titled *Getting to Yes: Negotiating Agreement Without Giving In* by Roger Fisher, Bruce M. Patton, and William L. Ury.[17] This book outlines methods to remove emotion from negotiations and separate people from the problem in an effort to gain a win-win situation.

To help maintain the value of a support function, such as patient education, it's paramount that patient education managers think strategically and talk the language of senior leaders. Without this skill, patient education becomes nothing more than a routine task performed by healthcare professionals at the bedside. Connecting the dots for administrators is crucial to the survival and future growth of patient education.

References

1. The Institute for Healthcare Improvement. "SBAR Technique for Communication: A Situational Briefing Model." The Institute for Healthcare Improvement Web site, *www.ihi.org/IHI/Topics/PatientSafety/SafetyGeneral/Tools/SBARTechniqueforCommunicationASituationalBriefingModel.htm* (accessed October 3, 2008).

2. The Institute of Medicine. "Report Brief. To Err is Human: Building a Safer Health System." The Institute of Medicine Web site, *www.iom.edu/CMS/8089/5575/4117.aspx* (accessed October 3, 2008).

3. Guise, N. "Do you speak SBAR?" *Journal of Gynecologic & Neonatal Nursing* 35 (2006): 313–314.

4. Value Based Management.net. "Rogers model for the adoption and diffusion of innovations." Value Based Management.net Web site, *www.valuebasedmanagement.net/methods_rogers_innovation_adoption_curve.html* (accessed October 4, 2008).

5. Fernsler, J., and Cannon, C. "The whys of patient education." *Seminars in Oncology Nursing* 7 (2001): 79–86.

6. The Patient Safety and Quality Improvement Act of 2005 (Public Law 109-41). The Agency for Healthcare Research and Quality Web site, *www.ahrq.gov/qual/psoact.htm* (accessed August 25, 2008).

7. American Society for Healthcare Risk Management. "An Overview of the Patient Safety Movement in Healthcare." *Plastic Surgical Nursing* 26 (2006): 116–120.

8. Clayman, M., Clayman, S., Steele, M., et al. "A review of the Florida Moratoria Data: What we have learned in 6 years and the need for continued patient education." *Annals of Plastic Surgery* 58 (2007):

9. Flippin, C. "Patient Safety through Patient Education in a Charity Medical Program." *Plastic Surgical Nursing* 26 (2006): 145–148.

10. Davis-Lenane, D., Hamilton, J., Gwozdz, J., et al. "Impact of the addition of patient education on the measurement of patient satisfaction." *Academy for Health Services Research and Health Policy Meeting.* 2000.

11. Brake, H., Sassmann, H., Noeres, D., Neiss, M., Geyer, S. "Ways to obtain a breast cancer diagnosis, consistency of information, patient satisfaction and the presence of relatives," *Support Care Cancer,* 15 (2007): 841–847.

12. Ronnberg, K., Lind, B., Zoega, B., Halldin, K., Gellerstedt, M., Brisby, H. "Patients' satisfaction with care/information and expectations on clinical outcome after lumbar disc herniation surgery," *Spine* 32(2) (2007): 256–261.

13. Oterhals, K., Hanestad, B.R., Eide, G.E., Hanssen, T.A. "The relationship between in-hospital information and patient satisfaction after acute myocardial infarction," *European Journal of Cardiovascular Nursing* 5(4) (2006): 303–310.

14. Krishel, S., Baraff, L.J. "Effect of emergency department information on patient satisfaction," *Annals of Emergency Medicine* 22 (1993): 568–572.

15. Centers for Medicare & Medicaid Services. "HCAHPS: Patients' Perspectives of Care Survey." Centers for Medicare & Medicaid Services Web site, *www.cms.hhs.gov/hospitalqualityinits/30_hospitalhcahps.asp* (accessed October 6, 2008).

16. Jha, A., Orav, J., Zheng, J., Epstein, A. "Patients' perception of hospital care in the United States," *The New England Journal of Medicine* 359 (2008). 1921–1931.

17. Fisher, R., Ury, W., Patton, B. *Getting to Yes: Negotiating Agreement Without Giving In*. Boston: Houghton Mifflin, 1992.

18. Agency for Healthcare Research and Quality. "Patient Safety Organizations." The Agency for Healthcare Research and Quality Web site, *www.pso.ahrq.gov/psos/overview.htm* (accessed November 10, 2008).

Engaging and Educating the Staff

A Challenging Arena

Engaging the frontline staff in patient education is probably one of the greatest challenges a patient education manager must face. The patient care environment is often plagued by such factors as a growing number of patients and inadequate number of staff members, while more expectations are continually being placed on healthcare providers. These additional expectations come from many different sources, including the following:

- Regulatory agencies that have updated standards for bedside care

- Internal initiatives that are being piloted on the units

- Orientation of new graduate nurses and the realities of short staffing, which result in overtime

In addition, patients and their families turn to many sources to obtain health information today, and therefore they are generally more informed when entering the healthcare system than they have been in the past. Often, patients feel they need to be informed beforehand so as to make the best use of their provider's time, as well as to act as their own advocate in a healthcare system that is fraught with errors. The Institute of Medicine's report, *To Err Is Human: Building a Safer Health System*, has been in the mainstream media, alerting patients to the dangers of healthcare. In addition, patients are increasingly turning to sources such as television and the Internet to obtain health information.[1] Patients going to the Internet in particular appear to be looking for information about the following:

- A condition

- Treatment

- Symptoms

- Advice about symptoms

- Advice about treatment[5]

Because patients tend to be entering the healthcare system already somewhat informed of their health status, clinical staff members, particularly nurses, need to be skilled in serving media-educated patients. We will discuss ways to accomplish this later in this chapter.

Nursing/staff ratios generally are challenging, and as we've just discussed, the average patient today has a much higher acuity level than in the past. With each new requirement or update in practice, more expectations are placed on nurses. The reality is that the bedside provider is faced with many challenges in accomplishing the basics of patient care and all the required documentation that accompanies such care. Therefore, nurses often view the amount of time they can devote to patient education as limited. I'd like to think this is because almost all bedside care providers want to take as much time as the patient needs to explain topics and truly evaluate comprehension, but they are faced with such time management challenges that patient education is reduced to patient teaching, a task to be checked off the task list as it is completed.

The irony is that, by virtue of healthcare becoming increasingly complex and patients' acuity levels rising, many patients are being sent home sicker and requiring more skills to maintain their health at home. Because of this, patient education is critical and must be delivered in an innovative way by staff members who are equipped to do so. In the past, patient education was modeled after a healthcare system that had patients with much longer lengths of stay. However, this approach was never updated to reflect the current environment, which advocates for shorter lengths of stay.[10]

The challenge to this begins with the allied health curriculum, particularly nursing. Depending on the decade in which a nurse was educated and his or her clinical experience, the expectations and framework for patient education vary. For instance, nurses who graduated in the 1970s were taught that all patient education begins with an anatomy and physiology lesson; a definite medical approach as opposed to a patient-centered approach.[10] In the 1980s, nurses were taught to focus their efforts on high-risk patients in a discharge planning framework.[10] And in the 1990s, nurses were taught to pare down patient education and to focus instead on "survival skills"—the skills a patient needs to stay safe at home.[10] Today, with health literacy and patient- and family-centered care viewed as a best practice in healthcare, nurses need to educate patients within all of these contexts.

 Effectively Managing Patient Education

This large variance in how nurses have been prepared to deliver patient education over the years likely means that your facility sees such variance as well. It's essential, therefore, to determine what standard of practice you want patient education to reflect in your organization, and to develop courses that will help to bridge this gap. Here are some ways to do this:

- Include a section in your patient care orientation documentation that describes the basics of patient education, how patient education should be delivered in your facility, and what tools are available to staff members to provide patient education, as well as how to access them

- Require an annual course, concurrent with other annual required courses, that reviews patient education basics and expectations for the clinical staff

- Offer optional patient education classes that focus on more specialized skills, such as writing materials and independently checking reading levels of patient education documents

The difficulty of measuring specific outcomes and documenting specific teaching interventions can be significantly challenging. Despite this, and the commonly held belief that "if it wasn't documented, it wasn't done," we all know patient education occurs all the time at the bedside. Every time a nurse enters a patient's room, hangs a new medication, and tells the patient what it is and what it's for—every time a nurse answers a question a patient has about his or her plan of care or clarifies a physician statement—education has taken place. Yet documentation is the weakest area within the patient education process.[3]

The Joint Commission requires several aspects of patient education to be documented, such as the following:

- The learning needs assessment

- Any barriers to learning

- Learning goals set by the care provider

- The information and skills taught

- Additional learning needs or follow-up needed

- Recommendations for different learning goals, if needed

- Revised goals, if necessary[4]

In addition to this, the location in which caregivers must document their education needs to be specific. If patient education is an interdisciplinary process/expectation at your facility, documentation needs to be interdisciplinary as well. And although many organizations have specific education flow sheets and do document education, often that documentation is lacking and does not coincide with the following points taken from The Joint Commission's *Guide to Patient & Family Education*:[4]

- The patient's full name needs to be recorded on every page of the documentation

- The date and time must be recorded on all documentation entries

- The caregiver must sign all entries

- Entries should be objective, specific, accurate, and truthful

- Entries need to be concise and comprehensive

- Entries must be documented in chronological order

For example, the following represents a good documentation note on patient education:

11/10/08 11:48 a.m. Patient instructed on how to self-administer insulin, including how to draw up medication in a syringe and select an injection site. Patient taught via verbal instruction, video, and "Insulin Administration" handout. Comprehension assessed via teach-back method. — J. Smith, RN

But there is a distinct difference between patient *teaching* and patient *education*. As patient education managers, we need to help staff members reframe what patient education is, and move it from a task to a process that is inherent in nursing. As noted by Fran London, MS, RN, in her book, *No Time to Teach?*, ". . . patient and family education goes beyond information . . . A nurse helps a patient interpret an illness and integrate that experience and its implications into his or her life."[9] This integration into daily living through which the nurse helps the patient is what makes patient education more than merely a task.

Engaging and educating staff members in patient education is a challenge that you need to tackle systematically, while recognizing the many obstacles that influence your ability to completely engage the staff. This chapter will discuss the steps involved in getting your arms around the current state of the bedside staff and targeting your staff development initiatives. Although no solution to the current challenges is perfect, this chapter will prepare the patient education manager to arrive at his or her own solutions.

Tackling Staff Development

The needs assessment

This necessary first step is often overlooked, but without the information from a needs assessment, you risk investing in a large initiative that may cover areas your staff members don't particularly require. This can result in wasted effort on your behalf, as well as the missasignment of pulling staff members from patient care duties to an inservice or staff development opportunity from which they will not achieve any type of measurable improvement. The needs assessment need not be terribly complex or lengthy; in fact, the more complex and lengthy it is, the less likely you will get the staff to fill out your survey. Rather, you need a good idea of what your staff members are thinking and feeling relative to patient education. You'll find an example of a needs assessment survey later in this chapter.

A needs assessment is a way to gather data that will help you define a problem that must be solved. You can gather data from a variety of sources, including your hospital administrators, clinical staff members, patients, current literature findings, and best practices, but the data should arise primarily from The Joint Commission's requirements for improvement (RFI), high-risk/high-volume concerns and diagnoses, and issues that affect patient safety.

It is critical to be a member of your hospital's patient safety committee, in addition to being involved in your hospital's Joint Commission/accreditation team. During meetings of such committees, information regarding your facility's performance on accreditation surveys is shared, including details concerning specifics that were cited. Also, by being a part of these committees, you can get a sense of what are considered to be high-risk/high-volume/problem-prone concerns at your facility. For example, if anticoagulation therapy is considered high-risk and high-volume at your facility, you should focus on this area, because patient safety is at greater risk in this than in other areas.

Staff members are gold mines of information that we often forget to use. Perhaps staff members are aware that patient education should represent more than merely giving a patient a handout, but patient care time is precious, and different priorities compete for that time, such as a new hospital initiative or protocols and requirements. Highlight for staff members, either in a patient education newsletter or in other educational offerings, the benefit of patient education and how it can actually save time. That notion may be hard for staff members to grasp, so the patient education manager needs to reframe thoughts regarding how patient education is delivered.

When patient education is viewed as a task, similar to starting an IV or giving a patient a bath, staff members naturally see it as "one more thing" they need to complete during their shift and another item they need to check off as having completed. They may not realize that the less time they spend educating their patients, the more likely it is that their patients will have additional questions and potentially use the call light.

For example, if a patient who is at risk for falling because of postanesthesia is not instructed on how to get out of bed properly and when to call for help, the patient may attempt to walk on his or her own, and may end up falling. As a result, the patient will get hurt and the nurse must stop what he or she is doing to respond to an urgent situation that could have been prevented. To avoid such scenarios, the patient education manager needs to communicate to staff members the need for patient education at every available opportunity, and particularly during education offerings.

Perhaps staff members have a hunger for more information about health literacy, or perhaps staff members don't understand how health literacy affects them and the care they provide to patients. Doing your homework to determine what information your staff wants and needs can help you fine-tune initiatives to engage them.

Creating a Staff Development Action Plan

Staff development is a major task, and many healthcare organizations employ educators and specialists to address this issue. As a patient education manager, you should rarely be alone in your staff development endeavors; instead, reach out to your staff development colleagues and tap into their wealth of knowledge and experience in this area. In this way, you can come prepared with a staff development action plan, complete with details regarding staff concerns and recommendations for the best ways to address them. See Figure 3.1 for a sample staff development action plan for patient education.

FIGURE 3.1   Staff development action plan for patient education

Need/goal	Supporting evidence	Intervention	Outcome	Evaluation method	Measure of success	Strategic goal link
Patient education needs to be documented in the medical record according to established standards	Joint Commission standard PC.02.03.01 RFI at last survey (October 2008) Hospital policy #5678 Chart audits reveal 50% compliance	Policy update and review Inservice for staff members	Patient education is documented according to standards	Chart audits Accreditation survey	90% compliance No RFIs	Quality
Patient education materials need to be written at a sixth-grade reading level	Joint Commission white paper on health literacy Institute for Healthcare Improvement recommendations	Policy creation Workshop for authors of patient education materials	Materials are written at or below a sixth-grade level Patients are able to understand their education information	Review all patient education materials prior to distribution Make a follow-up phone call to patients after discharge	90% of all patient education materials meet requirement Patients verbalize improved understanding	Patient-/family-centered care

Other things to do as you begin to determine staff development needs relative to patient education include the following:

- Conduct a brief survey of staff members to determine their interests (see Figure 3.2).

- Compare existing policies and procedures with what is actually occurring in practice. For example, if your policy about patient education states that care providers must evaluate patient understanding using the teach-back method, but you find that patient education is assessed by a patient signature, this may indicate a gap in knowledge.

- Conduct chart audits. How is patient education being documented? Is it meeting the Joint Commission standards for patient education documentation? Is it including essential elements such as what was taught, what teaching method was used, and the patient's response?

- Evaluate patient education materials authored and/or selected by staff members. Are they meeting readability requirements? If not, the staff may lack the skills to write patient-centered materials. As a rule, patient education handouts should be patient-friendly and meet readability criteria as established by the Suitability Assessment of Materials tool by Doak, Doak, and Root. (We'll discuss this tool in more detail in Chapter 4.)

The answers to these and other questions can help you to tailor your staff development initiatives and make the best use of time while achieving real outcomes.

FIGURE 3.2

Staff self-needs assessment

Please answer the following questions to help us determine patient and family education needs at our hospital. Thank you.

1. Please indicate which patient education topics you would like to know more about:
   a. Joint Commission standards _____
   b. Health literacy concepts _____
   c. Creating patient education materials _____
   d. Designing patient education programs _____
   e. Evaluating comprehension _____
   f. Other _____

2. About which of the following topics do your patients typically ask you for more information?
   a. Diseases/conditions
   b. Procedures
   c. Discharge instructions
   d. Medications

3. Do you feel you have the tools to answer your patients' questions appropriately?
   a. Yes
   b. No

4. If not, what tools do you need?_____

5. Please indicate anything else that may be helpful to you in educating your patients.
   _____
   _____
   _____
   _____

Thank you!

Innovative Learning Approaches: Solutions That Work

Given the difficulty in reaching the frontline staff for education inservices, it's necessary to think of innovative and engaging ways to get your message out and create learning experiences. Even the most interesting topics can be diluted with a very mundane and boring delivery. General adult education principles suggest that adults learn best when you use the following techniques:

- Make them feel like they have control of their learning and the method for acquiring new knowledge

- Make them feel respected for the life experiences and other knowledge they bring to the classroom

- Provide educational experiences that build on previous experiences and have relevance to staff members' daily work and/or life

- Use a variety of teaching methods, such as lectures combined with an interactive game, group work, discussion, and visuals

Essentially, the paradigm by which we all typically learn, the hour-long lecture, is the least effective way to reach your learners.

Using computer-based learning modules or tutorials can be of great advantage; creating programs that are online and interactive can promote staff education that is ". . . convenient, user-friendly and cost effective."[5] Not only does this type of education allow for a variety of teaching methods, but it also allows staff members to conveniently access the information in between patient care responsibilities, taps into various learning styles, and allows self-paced learning—all of which are consistent with adult learning principles.

One example that highlights the success achieved via this method is the work of Jackie Smith, associate professor, Clinical University of Utah College of Nursing, and Nancy Lombardo, systems librarian, Spencer S. Eccles Health Sciences Library University of Utah, who took a six-hour workshop on patient education and transformed it into a CD-ROM that allows users to self-pace and complete the workshop in a modular way. Preliminary evaluation findings of the program have been very positive.[5]

Train-the-Trainer methodologies tend to be used frequently; however, the effectiveness of this method for education hasn't been researched thoroughly in the literature, and I do not feel that this strategy will likely be the most effective. Rather, developing fun and interactive methods, such

Effectively Managing Patient Education

as games that another staff member or unit manager can administer at department meetings, is an innovative way to help foster learning. Chain Reaction,[6] a game that fosters learning about the National Patient Safety Goals, is a fun and interactive game designed to keep staff members on their toes while learning the elements of performance for each Goal. Although this game was developed within my organization to address the National Patient Safety Goals, you can adapt it for use with any content. A PowerPoint presentation on the CD-ROM included with this book contains a copy of the game and directions.

Another instructional method that appears to connect staff members with your content is storytelling. As educators, we are often focused on delivering our key objectives, but sometimes the best way to convey a point is through storytelling. For example, as part of a curriculum regarding health literacy, you may want to tell stories about how patients at your facility were unable to understand the materials they received, and, as a result, had to spend time calling other healthcare organizations to clarify the information. A great example of storytelling as an effective education method is the American Medical Association's 2007 video, *Health Literacy and Patient Safety: Help Patients Understand*, in which actual patients convey their stories regarding how low health literacy affected their healthcare. Staff members tend to respond very well to this type of learning and often request copies of the stories to share with others.

The curriculum for staff development programs is usually formed with the assistance of staff development educators, but generally, your objectives for any staff development program on patient education should touch on the following:

- Basics of patient education practices, such as the patient education process (see Figure 3.3).

- Specific requirements, as outlined in your institution's patient education policy.

- Issues that arise that signify a gap in practice (e.g., documentation issues as cited by a Joint Commission survey).

- Skills needed for nurses to respond to patients who are media-educated.[7] In particular, nurses need to step back and look at the medical information disseminated in the media today, and attempt to understand what a patient sees. Explore the information you find on television and in pop-culture magazines such as *Fitness, Shape, Cosmopolitan*, and *Prevention*. Search the Internet and become well-versed in what Web sites such as WebMD offer patients. It's prudent to know what tools and information your patients come equipped with so that you can better respond to their concerns and questions.

FIGURE 3.3 The patient education process

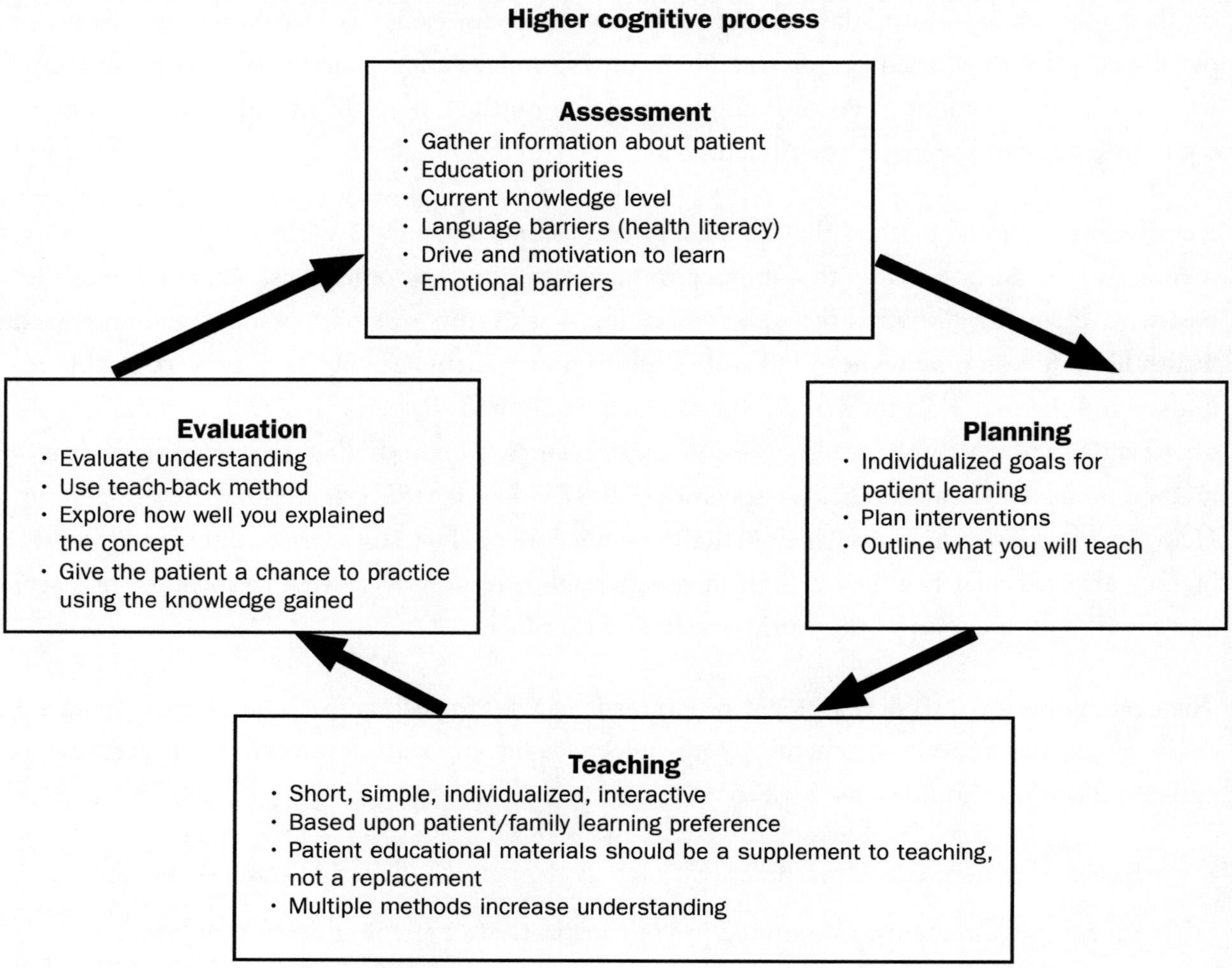

Higher cognitive process

Assessment
- Gather information about patient
- Education priorities
- Current knowledge level
- Language barriers (health literacy)
- Drive and motivation to learn
- Emotional barriers

Planning
- Individualized goals for patient learning
- Plan interventions
- Outline what you will teach

Evaluation
- Evaluate understanding
- Use teach-back method
- Explore how well you explained the concept
- Give the patient a chance to practice using the knowledge gained

Teaching
- Short, simple, individualized, interactive
- Based upon patient/family learning preference
- Patient educational materials should be a supplement to teaching, not a replacement
- Multiple methods increase understanding

Demonstrating that you know more than your patients is easy: teaching is more difficult.

—*The Practice of Patient Education*. Redman, B. (2006).

Effectively Managing Patient Education

Although patients are generally more informed today than ever before, it's important not to dismiss the information they find from pop-culture sources and the Internet. Be cautious, however; realize that not all information from these sources is reliable and credible (which is why you need to be familiar with what is out there), and provide your patients with ways to determine how they can know whether the information they find is credible. Instructing patients to look for information from reliable sources such as WebMD and the U.S. Centers for Disease Control and Prevention, as well as informing them of the importance of looking for copyright dates when utilizing any information to check for timeliness, can help patients without discouraging them from finding information on their own.

Navigating Through Negativity

As we discussed earlier in this chapter, many challenges exist in trying to engage the bedside staff in patient education. Since staff members can sometimes view patient education as being less important than other aspects of patient care, such as assessments, dressing changes, and other highly technical nursing skills, the burden rests with the patient education manager to promote patient education and demonstrate its importance in patient care. An excellent resource for both you and bedside staff members is the aforementioned book, *No Time to Teach?*, which speaks directly to the caregiver and explains not only how patient education is part and parcel of the nursing practice, but also how providing patient education can save nurses time. As noted in Chapter 2, when patient education is viewed not as a task, but rather as being integrated into the daily care nurses provide, a dynamic conversation can occur between the nurse and the patient, and individualized teaching, a hallmark characteristic of patient- and family-centered care, can occur.

Patient- and family-centered care is a concept that many professional organizations and regulatory agencies discuss; in fact, The Joint Commission is in the process of developing Culturally Competent and Patient-Centered Care Standards. Through a partnership with the Commonwealth Fund, The Joint Commission will develop these standards, which address the needs of patients from a cultural and patient-centered perspective. The project will address how to better incorporate culture, diversity, language, and health literacy issues into the existing Joint Commission standards or into the development of entirely new standards. The project is set to run through January 2010. You can find more detailed information regarding patient-/family-centered care in Chapter 4.

Reflecting back to Chapter 2, in which we discussed obtaining organizational support, you know that leadership engagement is crucial to forward movement and growth of an initiative or process. With that forward movement and growth, staff engagement can occur. When staff members resist change or are unable to see the imperative behind patient education (or any process), having senior leaders on board to champion (and at times, strongly recommend) their efforts can help. After all, if the chief nursing officer does not value patient education, why would his or her staff members?

As the patient education manager, conveying your passion for the field also helps to engage others. A great place to share your knowledge is the Health Care Education Association (HCEA). This professional organization, which comprises patients and other health educators, can provide you with a wealth of invaluable knowledge and expertise. Talk to others about patient education, show your enthusiasm, and share your research as though it's the most important topic in the world! Energy is contagious, so let yours flow. To find the HCEA Web site, visit *www.hcea-info.org*

Recognizing a Job Well Done

Conducting and hosting special events and programs are great ways to engage staff members, as well as to provide a forum for additional support for patient education. One method for doing this is to create patient education events to be held on key dates. Some of those observances include the following:

- **Health Literacy Month,** October 1–31: This annual event promotes the importance of clear health information and communication. Started by Helen Osborne in 1999, Health Literacy Month is a great time to launch new patient education staff development classes. I once used this occasion to unveil a much-desired writing workshop for staff members who were interested in learning how to apply health literacy principles in their development of patient education materials. See Figure 3.4 for a sample lesson plan.

- **National Health Education Week,** October 20–24: This week is designed to bring awareness to, and celebrate, the many ways that health education affects individual, community, and public health.

- **Patient Education Week,** fourth week of November: This week promotes patient education practices and their effect on health and safety, and celebrates the contributions patient educators make to the health and well-being of others. This can be a great opportunity to showcase recent advancements in patient education at your organization.

FIGURE 3.4 | Sample lesson plan for health literacy month

Lesson Plan
Writing for Patients and Families Workshop

Intended audience: All staff members who write correspondence or education for patients, their families, and the community

Total class time (including one 15-minute break): 4 hours

Purpose:
1. Provide staff members with the knowledge and skills necessary to write easy-to-understand and easy-to-read patient and family correspondence
2. Help speed up the approval process of patient education materials

Objectives:
1. Discuss how low health literacy affects health outcomes.
2. Incorporate key elements of plain-language principles when developing patient education material.
3. Discuss how to produce materials that score a "superior" rating on the Suitability Assessment of Materials (SAM) tool.
4. Describe the process for developing patient education materials.

Registration: iLearning

Preclass student assignment: Come prepared with a draft of a patient education or correspondence document; read David Ausabel's theory of subsumption at *http://tip.psychology.org/ausubel.html.*

Assumptions:

Equipment:
1. Folder with writing reference guide, process flow sheet, evaluation form, SAM tool, book list
2. Computer and projector
3. Whiteboard/chalkboard

FIGURE 3.4   Sample lesson plan for health literacy month (cont.)

Evaluation:
- Documents at a sixth-grade reading level
- Patient education documents scoring a "superior" rating on the SAM tool at first evaluation
- Faster approval process

Other methods to educate systemwide:

Method	Topic	Owner	Completion due date	Comments

Time	Topic	Content	Learning activities	Media/AV
45 min.	General literacy Health literacy	• Introduction • Definition • Statistics • Solutions	Didactic	PowerPoint video
60 min.	Begin your writing project Clear writing techniques	• Getting started • Identifying your audience • Defining objectives • Making an outline Principles: • Writing style (second versus third person) • Active versus passive voice • Language consistency • Reader engagement • Content: behavior versus fact; limited scope; advance organizers (subsumption theory) • Plain words • Writing at a sixth-grade level • Sequencing of information • Simple versus complex sentences	Didactic Case studies	PowerPoint whiteboarding

Effectively Managing Patient Education

FIGURE 3.4   Sample lesson plan for health literacy month (cont.)

20 min.	Overview of read-ability tools	SMOG Flesch-Kincaid Fry	Didactic	
20 min.	Submitting and publishing your work	Overview of the patient education development process		
30 min.	Getting to know the SAM tool	Overview of the SAM tool; Understanding what the SAM tool measures	Review SAM tool; grade the pre-class assign-ment with the SAM tool; discuss	
30 min.	Summary			

Additional tools created from project:

Providing patient education awards is also a fun way to promote patient education, as well as offering an opportunity to celebrate staff members' efforts. You can confer awards for materials or programs developed, or for a patient interaction that highlighted the best practices of patient education. See Figure 3.5 for a sample award form. Bedside caregivers are receptive to public recognition, and they often view that as being more desirable than small tokens or gifts. In fact, public recognition events have been recognized as promising practices for engaging the nursing work force.[10]

Effective patient education requires the engagement of frontline staff members who educate patients directly, in the form of bedside teaching, formal classes, and/or community programs. Because many healthcare disciplines provide patient education, yet few have received formal training,[3] it's important that the patient education manager take steps to provide ongoing development in this area.

FIGURE 3.5   Sample patient education award form

Patient Education Award Nomination Form

Please route to the patient education committee by September 1.

Have you witnessed an exemplary patient education practice, in the form of materials, programs, patient interactions, or documentation? Nominate your fellow staff member via this form! Self-nominations are also accepted.

Nominee's name: _____Extension: _____

Your name (if different from the nominee): _____Extension: _____

Check in which category the staff member is being nominated:
- ❏ Materials (written/video/Web-based)—*please submit a sample*
- ❏ Programs/classes—*please submit curriculum/lesson plan*
- ❏ Events
- ❏ Documentation—*please submit charting*
- ❏ Patient—provider interaction

Please describe why you are nominating this individual and why his or her work exemplifies patient education best practices.

_____

_____

_____

_____

_____

_____

Thank you for your submission! The patient education committee will carefully review your nomination. The nominee's education record and his or her attendance at patient education programs will be considered with the nomination.

Award recipients will be notified via phone and will be honored at the Annual Patient Education Awards Breakfast.

References

1. Shuyler, K., and Knight, K. "What are patients seeking when they turn to the Internet? Analysis of questions asked by visitors to an Orthopaedics Web Site." *Journal of Medical Internet Research* 5 (2003): 5.

2. Kruger, S. "The patient educator role in nursing." *Applied Nursing Research* 4 (1991): 19–24.

3. Djonne, M. "Development of a core competency program for patient educators." *Journal for Nurses in Staff Development* 23 (2007): 155.

4. The Joint Commission. *The Joint Commission Guide to Patient and Family Education.* Oakbrook Terrace, IL: *Joint Commission Resources,* 2003.

5. Smith, J., and Lombardo, N. "Patient education workshop on CD-ROM." *Journal for Nurses in Staff Development* 21 (2005): 46.

6. Smith, T. "Chain Reaction Board Game." ProHealth Care. 2008.

7. Herzberger, S. "Nursing media-educated patients." *Journal for Nurses in Staff Development* 24 (2008): 101–104.

8. The Advisory Board Company. "Engaging the Nurse Workforce: Best Practices for Promoting Exceptional Staff Performance." *www.advisory.com* (accessed October 7, 2008).

9. London, F. *No Time to Teach? A Nurse's Guide to Patient and Family Education.* Philadelphia: Lippincott Williams & Wilkins, 1999.

10. Rankin, S., and Stallings, K. *Patient Education: Principles & Practice, 4th ed.* Philadelphia: Lippincott, 1991.

Bibliography

Avillion, A. *A Practical Guide to Staff Development: Tools and Techniques for Effective Education.* Marblehead, MA: HCPro, Inc., 2004.

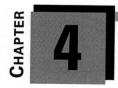
The Pillars of Patient Education

The Pillars of Excellent Patient Education

As discussed in previous chapters, patient education has broad implications that span many areas:

- Satisfaction among patients and staff members

- Improved patient safety

- Positive health outcomes

- Accomplishment of organizational strategic goals

As a result, it's important to recognize what I consider to be the four pillars of patient education (see Figure 4.1):

- Health literacy

- Patient-centered care

- Language

- Culture

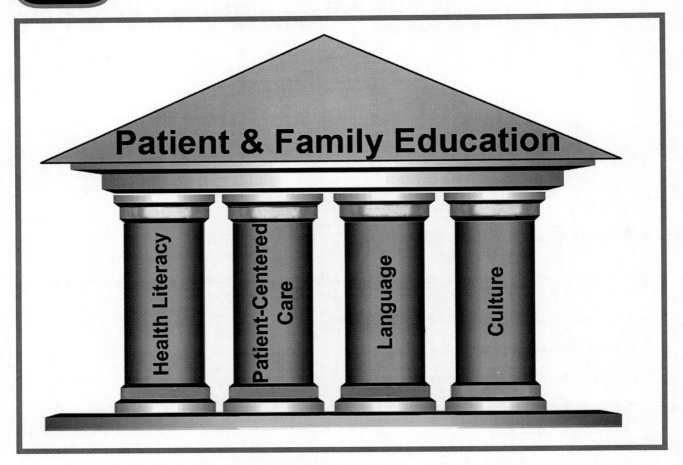

FIGURE 4.1 Pillars of patient education

These four pillars are the main building blocks of any solid patient education endeavor, be it a one-on-one interaction between a nurse and a patient or an organizational level initiative. Without these foundational pillars, patient education falls short of being a comprehensive and coordinated approach and places patients at risk.

Imagine, for example, the following scenarios:

- **Scenario 1:** A 28-year-old single mother is with her 2-year-old child, who was admitted for dehydration resulting from an upper respiratory infection. The mother dropped out of school in the sixth grade. The nurse provides the mother with some handouts on dehydration and fever management that are written at a twelfth-grade reading level, tells the mother that these handouts provide all the information she needs to know to care for her daughter, and walks out of the exam room.

 Effectively Managing Patient Education

- **Scenario 2:** A 44-year-old man who was recently diagnosed with diabetes mellitus is afraid of needles, and is very concerned that he will have to administer his own injections. When the nurse enters his room, he relays his fear and concern to her. The nurse responds by instructing the patient on the physiology of diabetes, because she believes the foundation for diabetes education is to understand how the illness works.

- **Scenario 3:** The senior executives of Community Healthcare and Hospitals are in a budget meeting, discussing various initiatives that require funding for implementation. One of the initiatives is a translation service that will provide large-volume translations for health education materials given to patients; currently, materials are available only in English, despite the fact that the Spanish-speaking population of patients at the facility is rising. The funding for this initiative is denied in favor of a larger budget for information services.

- **Scenario 4:** A couple brings their newborn into the emergency department. The parents are of Hmong descent, and do not speak English. They normally do not receive medical care from hospitals, but rather rely on herbs and other Hmong medicine practices. They have brought their infant in because their normal methods are not working. Doctors prescribe medications for the infant; however, the parents are upset by the side effects and feel strongly that the medications may permanently damage their infant's soul. The doctors are extremely frustrated that the parents will not follow orders, and as a result, the infant's condition worsens.

Each scenario demonstrates how patient education, at both the bedside and the leadership level, fails because one (or more) of the pillars is not taken into account or addressed. Although all of these scenarios are different, they have one thing in common: Patient education was provided, but ironically, it wasn't received. The differences between *providing* patient education and *receiving* education are drastic.

In all of the aforementioned scenarios, the patient education process was not utilized completely. Caregivers provided education that the patient didn't want/need to know (assessment and planning); caregivers didn't provide education in a way that the patient could understand (implementation); or caregivers did not fully assess what the patient learned from the interaction (evaluation). The only way to truly ensure that patient education has occurred is to use the "teach-back" evaluation method. Giving a patient a handout or even verbal instruction and simply asking "Do you understand?" is not effective in terms of evaluating patient understanding. How many times do caregivers receive a "no" response to that question? I have *never* had a patient answer "no" when I asked whether the patient understood what I just taught him or her. Yet I don't believe that every single patient I have cared for and instructed has walked away with a complete understanding of his or her instructions. I didn't realize it at the time, but I know it now. This is the critical difference between *providing* patient education and *receiving* patient education.

In the first scenario, the nurse provided patient education materials to the patient, but the nurse did not take the patient's health literacy into consideration. As a result, the mother will not understand what she needs to do to help keep her toddler healthy—she did not receive adequate patient education. This scenario also demonstrates the importance of educating families and highlights the role they play in caring for their loved ones. In this case it's obvious that the toddler was much too young to understand and to provide for her own hydration needs to effectively combat her dehydration. Here, the parent was the primary target for patient education.

Particularly in pediatrics, parents respond best to education that addresses their areas of concern.[20] In some instances the parent's area of concern is not necessarily what is considered medically to be a high priority, but you will not be very successful in educating a parent until you address his or her area of concern. So, for example, if a parent is concerned about his or her child's height/weight, but medically, the parent needs to be educated about a new diagnosis and how to manage it, it would be prudent to address the height/weight concerns first so that the parent can have those issues resolved, and then to move on to other topics that are also important.

In the second scenario, the nurse provided education to the patient, but she did not take into account the patient's concern or fear relative to the new diagnosis, particularly having to administer an injection by himself. The entire encounter was nurse-directed, as opposed to patient-centered, which could mean the patient's readiness to learn is lacking. If the patient is distracted by the thought of having to self-administer insulin, he is not going to process an anatomy and physiology lesson on diabetes. In addition, is anatomy and physiology really what the patient wants and needs to know? Moving from nurse-directed to patient-centered communication takes practice, and often role-playing is the best way to hone the skill and understand its effect on patient education outcomes.

In the third scenario, it can reasonably be assumed that patient education is being provided appropriately and on a routine basis within the hospital. What is lacking, however, are appropriate written materials for the increasing number of non–English–speaking patients that the hospital routinely admits. Given that the Decision was made *not* to fund a translation service to provide materials in Spanish, or other languages non–English–speaking patients will not have the appropriate patient education materials and will likely understand very little, if any, information provided to them in English. How effective is patient education when the patient doesn't read the language in which it's provided?

In the last scenario, the patient's condition worsened when the caregiver failed to address the patient's culture and her family's approach to medicine. The caregiver certainly provided education, but not within the appropriate cultural context, thereby allowing fear, misconception, and distrust to dominate.

All four of these examples demonstrate how patient education practices can collapse when they are not supported by the four pillars. Unfortunately the collapse is not obvious to the nurse at the bedside or to the senior executives in the board room. The collapse is insidious, particularly at the exact moment that a patient or his or her family members realize they do not understand an aspect of the patient's care, which is felt only by that patient and/or his or her family. The effects of the collapse can vary widely, but all of them distill to the common denominator of putting patients at risk.

It's critical that every patient education manager be knowledgeable about the four pillars, as well as how they are fundamental to patient education and how they intersect at all levels of patient care. This chapter will discuss the pillars in detail, along with strategies to address them in all of your patient education planning.

Health Literacy

Imagine you are trying to find a restaurant in a foreign city. You're driving in strange territory and realize you're lost. To find your way, you need access to some reliable information, and you need to be able to read, interpret, and apply that information. The information might be available on a map, but a map can be hard to understand, particularly if it's in small print. You could stop and ask for directions, but that will work only if the person you ask can provide you with the information you need in a clear and accurate way, and besides, you're too embarrassed to ask for directions anyway. Instead, you try to find your way as best you can through unknown streets, with signs you can't read or understand. This is what it's like to live with low health literacy while trying to navigate your way through the healthcare environment.

Overview and epidemiology

Health literacy has many formal definitions, but a widely accepted definition is that health literacy is the ability to read, understand, and act on health information. Low health literacy is a growing concern in healthcare and is estimated to affect up to 90 million people in the United States.[1] This means one in three patients who are seen or admitted into the hospital are likely to have low health literacy, and it's highly likely that they will be unable to understand most of the medical information and patient education put before them. Health information is essential to a patient's well-being and is directly linked to patient outcomes. In fact, literacy skills are a stronger predictor of health than age, income, employment status, education level, or racial/ethnic group.[2] Basically, low health literacy crosses all boundaries and does not discriminate. The disparities for population groups that already are considered vulnerable, such as racial/ethnic minorities and the elderly, are intensified when low health literacy comes into play. Studies show that low health literacy further widens the gap in these populations.[3]

The statistics for low health literacy continue to be alarming. Out of the 90 million American adults who have difficulty reading, 40 million to 44 million are considered functionally illiterate,[3] which means they are unable to perform basic reading tasks, such as reading the front page of a newspaper, a bus schedule, or directions for a microwave meal. Fifty million are considered marginally illiterate,[3] which means they have difficulty completing forms; these are the patients in the waiting room who begin to get anxious when presented with that dreaded clipboard containing forms they must fill out. As for the rest of America, the average reading skill of adults living in the United States is between eighth-and ninth-grade levels;[3] yet most healthcare information and patient education materials are communicated at a twelfth-grade level or beyond. These statistics demonstrate a very real crisis in healthcare today.

Health literacy also received the attention of The Joint Commission in its white paper, *What Did the Doctor Say? Improving Health Literacy to Protect Patient Safety*,[4] which contains several key recommendations for organizations to address health literacy, namely:

- Make effective communication a priority

- Address patients' communication needs across the care continuum

- Make policy changes that support/promote improved provider–patient communications

Specific details regarding how to operationalize those recommendations are contained within the white paper, which is available free of charge on the Joint Commission Web site (*www.jointcommission.org*)

A common question many caregivers ask regarding low health literacy is, "What about my patients who I know can read well and are educated professionals? Won't I insult their intelligence by 'talking down to them'?" The answer to this question is a resounding *no*. Numerous studies have documented that low health literacy can also affect seemingly literate patients. It's important to remember that even as educated professionals, these people are often confronted

Effectively Managing Patient Education

with unfamiliar terms and an unfamiliar environment when they are admitted to the hospital or are accompanying a loved one who is having health issues. The patient may not be feeling well, may be quite sick, and/or may be worried about his or her health status or that of his or her loved one, and in such cases, studies have shown that even very literate patients benefit from and appreciate simple communication.

Effect on Healthcare

The effect of low health literacy on the healthcare industry is even more sobering. As far as costs, patients with low health literacy have annual healthcare costs that are *four times higher* than those with higher literacy skills.[5] This can be attributed to patients simply being unable to understand what they need to do for follow-up care: what to do at home, how to take care of themselves, when to call the doctor, and/or how to take their medication. If a newly diagnosed diabetic patient has low health literacy, the likelihood that he or she will leave the hospital fully understanding how and when to check blood sugar, and what to do with certain blood sugar readings, is very low. As a result, these types of patients are susceptible to exacerbations of their condition, frequent readmissions, and overutilization of the emergency department. We know that only about 50% of all patients take their medications as directed;[6] could this be as a result of low health literacy? In fact, recent studies suggest that people with low health literacy make more medication errors[7] and are less able to comply with treatments.[2] Basically, low health literacy is a serious patient safety concern.

To better understand how low health literacy affects patient safety, examine James Reason's Swiss Cheese Model of Accident Causation[8] (also sometimes referred to as the cumulative act effect), which gives a great visual explanation of how an accident can occur despite defenses being in place. In Reason's model, each slice of Swiss cheese represents a barrier or protective mechanism that is designed to prevent an accident from occurring. The holes in the cheese represent latent failures that can occur; when those align, the end result is an accident, or, in the case of health-care, patient harm. This also demonstrates that addressing health literacy goes beyond ensuring that your materials are readable; it speaks to how staff members interact with patients, how welcoming the hospital environment is, and how well patient preferences are integrated into their care plan. See Figure 4.2 for an example of the Swiss Cheese model displayed in graphic form.

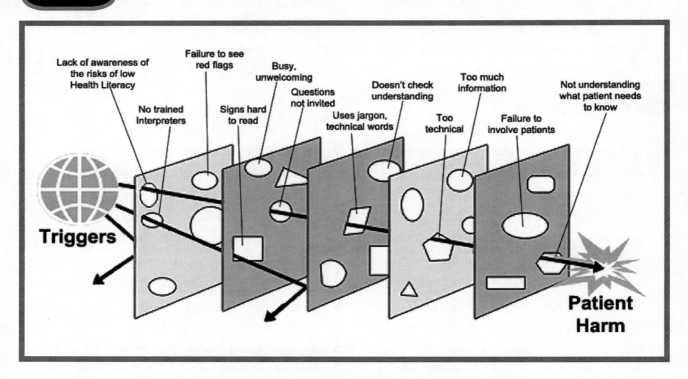

FIGURE 4.2 Reason's Swiss Cheese model of accident causation

Effective methods for making your care environment welcoming are simple to implement and include such acts as smiling when a patient or visitor approaches you or the front desk or displaying simple signs with phrases such as "How Can We Help?" Including patients in developing their plan of care is another great way to establish trust and convey an air of helpfulness and openness.

Assessing health literacy

One of the more common questions I receive from practitioners once they learn about health literacy is: "Is there a way for me to assess whether my patient has low health literacy?" The answer to that is yes. Unfortunately, however, many patients who have difficulty reading (and who often have low health literacy as a result) have spent their lives actively hiding their affliction from just about everyone with whom they come in contact. Being illiterate, particularly as an adult, can create embarrassing situations, and such patients will not tell anyone, let alone their healthcare provider, that they cannot read. These patients have learned how to cope with not being able to read, and have become skilled in hiding their problem. However, certain red-flag behaviors[9] indicate that a person may have difficulty reading, and thus is prone to low health literacy. These are:

 Effectively Managing Patient Education

- "Forgetting" his or her glasses and needing to read materials at home

- Opening pill bottles to identify medication, as opposed to reading the label

- Having his or eyes quickly

- Taking a long time to complete forms

- Requesting friends/family members in the room during patient education interactions

In addition to these red-flag behaviors, a few screening tools designed for use in the healthcare setting are also useful in assessing health literacy in a quantifiable way. You can find copies of these screening tools on the Internet; most are public domain and often are free to use. Three such screening tests come to mind: the Test of Functional Health Literacy in Adults, the Rapid Estimate of Adult Literacy in Medicine, and the Newest Vital Sign. All three tests are quick-assessment tools (less than three minutes) that clinicians can administer to determine at the bed-side the reading grade level of their patients.

Most screening tests require that the patient read aloud a set of words that are commonly found in healthcare materials; a certain scoring mechanism is in place to subsequently estimate what the patient's reading grade level would be. But what should the clinician do with the information obtained from these screening tools? Many experts, particularly those who developed the tools, recommend using these tools only for research purposes and only in aggregate form, as opposed to assessing individual patients. These screening tools have proven useful in the research arena, but you could make a case for utilizing the tools within your facility to aggregate data on the specific population you are serving to develop action plans to address needs.

A commonly held belief is that patients who have difficulty reading—and thus have low health literacy—are embarrassed to admit to this gap, and might find the thought of taking a reading comprehension test stressful. In addition, being sick and in the hospital, and in an unfamiliar environment, may already place stress on the patient; adding to that stress by assessing his or her reading skills may not be in the patient's best interests.

Finally, would the outcome of a health literacy screen really change the care a patient receives? The answer to that question is debatable. The scenarios I described earlier in this chapter identified how care was affected when the caregiver did not take health literacy into consideration. We then could assume that information from a health literacy screening would be useful in the care setting, as providers would adjust care based on the results, similar to how they would if they found out a patient had high blood pressure or high cholesterol.

However, similar to universal precautions regarding gowning and gloving to prevent the spread of infection among patients, if *all* patients are treated equally and if "universal precautions" relative to healthcare communication are utilized, screening patients for low health literacy becomes unnecessary. We do not actively screen all patients for infections before putting on gloves when providing direct patient care; yet we assume that all patients are potentially infectious, and to stop the spread of infection, we don gloves. With communication, if we assume that all patients can benefit from clear communication and we employ "universal precautions" for clear health communications, the need for screening every individual patient loses merit.

All of these valid discussion points regarding the use of screening tools in health literacy are compounded by a recent study that found that patients are *willing* to undergo literacy assessments during routine office visits, and that these assessments did not decrease their satisfaction with their care.[10] It's important to note that this is the only study on this subject; no other studies exist that can conclusively recommend whether screening is beneficial. Until patients' reactions to health literacy screening are fully understood, staying cognizant of low health literacy, being keenly aware of red flags, when interacting with patients, and continuously adjusting communication techniques to fit each patient are effective ways to deal with low health literacy.

Strategies for addressing low health literacy

Teaching Patients with Low Literacy Skills,[3] by Cecilia C. Doak, Leonard G. Doak, and Jane H. Root, is an excellent resource for patient education managers and clinicians alike. It discusses practical strategies regarding written materials, incorporating visuals, technology, learner verification, and general tips on teaching.

The Suitability Assessment of Materials (SAM) tool, developed by Doak, Doak, and Root, is the standard by which all patient education materials should be evaluated. Readability formulas have been used since the 1920s, and were used for the following seven decades prior to the development of SAM.[3] But measuring how easy a document is to read goes beyond determining the document's reading-grade level. Think about documents you come into contact with every day, such as billing statements, credit card statements, open enrollment information from your employer, and others. What makes those documents easy to read? Is it the font size? Is it how the information is organized on the page? Is it the use (or lack) of pictures and images? The readability of a document takes into account all of those factors, and more.

Figures 4.3, 4.4, and 4.5 show examples of patient education materials that are considered to score a superior rating on the SAM tool. Note the amount of white space on the page, the font

 Effectively Managing Patient Education

size, and the question-and-answer format, which fosters reader interaction. All these factors improve the readability of patient education materials.

FIGURE 4.3   Example of easy-to-read patient education document: Dental emergencies

Dental emergencies

Tooth injury (loosened, chipped, or knocked out)
Teeth that have been loosened, chipped, or pushed out of place need to be seen by a dentist and may need repositioning and stabilization. Permanent teeth that are knocked out are considered an emergency. Baby teeth that are knocked out can't be put back into place, but the underlying teeth need to be checked for damage.

What should I do if a permanent tooth is knocked out?
Gently rinse off the tooth with saliva or water. Do not scrub the tooth. If you are old enough and mature enough not to swallow the tooth, put the tooth back in the socket, facing the correct way. Bite down on a wad of cloth to keep the tooth in position until you can see a dentist.

What if I can't put the tooth back in?
Put the tooth in milk and get to a dentist right away. Do not leave the tooth dry or in tap water. This will damage the tooth within minutes.

Toothache
A toothache is pain in or around a tooth. Some reasons for a toothache include:
- Tooth decay (cavity)
- An infected tooth
- Infected gums
- An irritated tooth nerve
- A problem with the sinuses or jaw
- A fracture or crack in the tooth
- A damaged filling in the tooth
- Any injury that may have bruised a tooth

Tooth pain may be sharp, throbbing, or constant. Sometimes it may hurt only when you put pressure on the tooth. Cold or heat may worsen the pain. You may have swelling around the tooth or get a fever or headache.

FIGURE 4.3   Example of easy-to-read patient education document:
Dental emergencies (cont.)

Because a toothache can have a variety of causes, the best way to treat a toothache is to see your dentist. Generally, you can wait to go to the dentist until the next available appointment.

What to do for a toothache:
- Rinse the mouth with warm water to clean it out.
- Use dental floss to remove any food that might be trapped between the teeth.
- Put an ice pack on the jaw for 20 minutes.
- Swish warm saltwater around in the mouth. This can help reduce gum swelling.
- Put some oil of cloves on a small piece of cotton and place the cotton on the affected tooth. Keep the oil of cloves off the tongue because it stings.
- Do not place aspirin on the aching tooth or gum tissues.
- Take Tylenol or Motrin, following the directions on the bottle.

Dental abscess
A dental abscess is an infection from a germ (bacteria) around the root of a tooth. The infection may spread to the gums or jawbone. Some causes of dental abscesses are:

- Tooth decay
- Injury to a tooth, such as a severe blow to the tooth or jaw

In some cases, the cause of the abscess may not be known.

The infection causes pus to collect, creating a lump. You may have a fever or a red and swollen cheek or gums. If you have a lump, it may feel hot. Your tooth or mouth may hurt.

What are the symptoms of a dental abscess?
- Sensitivity to heat or cold
- A lingering ache
- Pain or throbbing with or without biting or chewing
- Redness and swelling of the gums
- Discolored teeth
- Tender glands in the neck
- A swollen face
- A bad taste in the mouth
- An open, draining sore on the side of the gums

FIGURE 4.3   **Example of easy-to-read patient education document: Dental emergencies (cont.)**

How is a dental abscess treated?
- Take antibiotics ordered by your doctor
- Rinse your mouth three to four times a day with warm saltwater
- Use an ice pack for 15 to 20 minutes every hour
- Brush at least twice a day and floss every day
- Take ibuprofen, acetaminophen, or another pain-relief medication as ordered by your dentist or doctor

How do I prevent a toothache?
The best way to prevent a toothache is to prevent damage to your teeth. Brush after every meal with a fluoride toothpaste, and floss your teeth. Additional safeguards include the following:

- See your dentist every six months.
- Follow a healthy diet for good dental health. Avoid foods with sugars, such as sweets and white bread, and sweet, sticky foods.

FIGURE 4.4   **Example of easy-to-read patient education document: Giving insulin**

Giving insulin

How should I choose an injection site?
- Injections are given in a layer of fat just below the skin.
- Four main sites can be used:
  - Abdomen (belly); this is the preferred site
  - Back of the upper arm; use only if someone else is giving you the injection
  - Front and upper, outer side of the thighs
  - Upper part of the buttocks
- Make sure you stay at least 2 inches away from the belly button.
- Avoid areas with scars or stretch marks.
- It is important to use a new spot (within the same body region) each time you give an injection. Move about 1 inch away from the previous injection site.

How do I draw up and give insulin?
1. Wash hands with soap and water.
2. Clean the top of the insulin bottle with alcohol.
3. Pull the plunger of the syringe back to _____units of air (equal to your insulin dose).
4. Stick the needle into the bottle and inject the air into the insulin bottle.
5. Leave the needle in the bottle and turn the bottle upside down.
6. Pull the plunger of the syringe back to _____ units of insulin.
7. Take the syringe out of the bottle.
8. Pinch a fold of the skin and inject the needle at a 90-degree angle (straight in).
9. Push the plunger into the syringe.
10. Discard the used syringe as directed by your local waste management company (**do not put the syringe in the regular garbage**).

What is the best way to care for my insulin?
- Check the expiration date on the bottle of insulin. Do not use the insulin if it is past the expiration date.
- Do not freeze the insulin.
- Once the bottle of insulin has been opened, you may keep it at room temperature for up to 30 days.
- Keep the insulin away from direct sunlight and heat sources.
- Always have extra bottles of insulin on hand and keep them in the refrigerator.
- Inspect the bottle of insulin before using. Only NPH and premixed insulin should be cloudy.

     Effectively Managing Patient Education

FIGURE 4.5 **Example of easy-to-read patient education document: Insurance coverage**

Insurance coverage

The staff at [Hospital name] would like to tell you some important information about your insurance coverage and doctor visits.

What do you need to do?
- Look at your insurance policy before your annual doctor visit.
- Tell your doctor of any rules during your visit.
- Call your insurance agent, your employer, or the Medicare benefits line at [phone number] if you have any questions.

What should you know?
- Once your doctor sees you and a diagnosis is made, the diagnosis cannot be changed. Changing it is against the law.
- You may have to come in for second office visit to talk about issues not addressed in your yearly visit.

If you request diagnostic consultation or treatment for a problem requiring additional time and diagnostic evaluation not addressed by a routine physical, you may be charged for another office visit.

We thank you for choosing us to meet your healthcare needs. It is our goal to provide excellent and thorough care to you as efficiently as possible.

Please call our business office at [phone number] if you have questions about our business policy.

[Hospital name] physicians and staff

As mentioned earlier, once clinicians learn about health literacy, there is a strong desire to iden-tify patients with low health literacy in an effort to provide targeted, individualized education for a particular skill level. Although this desire is noble, it has one major error: assuming that *only* those patients with difficulty reading would benefit from simplified health information. Although those patients certainly would benefit, even patients with high literacy skills benefit from and appreciate simpler health communication.[3]

Think about your own healthcare experiences: Although you may be a clinician by profession, when your child is the one in the emergency department, do you really want to put on your nurse's hat and interpret and sort through medical information to find out what's wrong with him or her? Or do you simply want to be a parent and be there to comfort your child while the nurses and physicians provide information to you in a clear and consistent manner? Most people would choose the latter option.

Therefore, approaching all patients with to clear communication techniques is the recommended method to ensure that all patients leave with the information they need to know in order to care for themselves or their loved one. Figure 4.6 outlines some general principles of clear communica-tion techniques.

FIGURE 4.6 Examples of clear communication techniques

Principle	Explanation	Example
Use a personal, conversational writing style.	Use second person as opposed to third person.	Use "you" or "your doctor" as opposed to "the doctor."
Use active voice. Passive voice is harder to comprehend.	Writing in active voice means the agent or doer of the action is the subject. Active sentences follow the agent-verb-receiver format.	Active: "Wash your hands before each meal." Passive: "Hands should be washed before each meal."
Be consistent in the terminology used.	Avoid confusing the reader by using several different terms for the same thing. Pick one and use it throughout.	Pick one term—for example, pills, medicine, or medication—rather than using all three in the same document.
Use common, one- and two-syllable words; define all medical terms.	Using one- to two-syllable words helps bring down the reading level.	Use "doctor" instead of "physician" and "pills" instead of "medication."
Engage the reader.	Documents that engage the reader are more likely to be read entirely and remembered.	Use a question-and-answer format or leave spaces for patients to fill in their responses on what they need to do.

Educating your organization about health literacy can be an overwhelming job, but there are many resources for you to turn to. Among them are the following:

- Health Literacy Consulting, *www.healthliteracy.com/*

- National Patient Safety Foundation and Ask Me 3, *www.npsf.org/askme3/*

- Agency for Healthcare Research and Quality Web site for health literacy and cultural competency, *www.ahrq.gov/browse/hlitix.htm*

- AMA Foundation health literacy kit, *www.ama-assn.org/ama/pub/category/9913.html*

The AMA Foundation has an excellent training kit that includes a video geared toward physicians, with vignettes from actual patients who relay their low health literacy experiences in the healthcare system. This video appeals to all audiences, but especially to physicians who tend to find value in information from other physicians.

Patient- and Family-Centered Care

Patient- and family-centered care is often described as an innovative approach to patient care, but once clinicians are familiar with what it means, most agree that it's simply the right thing to do. And arguably, the core concepts of patient- and family-centered care are central to many healthcare disciplines, particularly nursing. Patient- and family-centered care is grounded in a collaborative relationship with patients and their families, in which providers treat them holistically and actively involve them in all aspects of care. Although many different models of patient-centered care exist, a commonly held standard is that from the Institute for Family-Centered Care.

The Institute was founded in 1992 as a nonprofit, private organization dedicated to providing leadership and policy on the concepts and practice of patient- and family-centered care. Its mission, as defined on its Web site (*www.familycenteredcare.org*), is as follows:

> *In partnership with patients, families, and health care professionals from many disciplines, the Institute for Family-Centered Care promotes the understanding and practice of patient- and family-centered care. The Institute seeks to ensure that principles of patient- and family-centered care are reflected in all systems providing care and support to individuals and families, including health, education, mental health, and social services.*

In addition, the Institute has defined the core concepts of patient-/family-centered care as follows:

- **Dignity and respect:** Healthcare practitioners listen to and honor the patient's and his or her family's perspectives and choices. The knowledge, values, beliefs, and cultural backgrounds of the patient and his or her family are incorporated into the planning and delivery of care.

- **Information-sharing:** Healthcare practitioners communicate and share complete and unbiased information with patients and their families in ways that are affirming and useful. Patients and their families receive timely, complete, and accurate information to effectively participate in care and decision-making.

- **Participation:** Patients and their families are encouraged to participate in care and decision-making at the level they choose and supported for doing so.

- **Collaboration:** Patients and their families are consulted on an institutionwide basis. Healthcare leaders collaborate with patients and their families in policy and program development, implementation, and evaluation; in healthcare facility design; and in professional education, as well as in the delivery of care.[11]

Not only is patient education woven into all of these core concepts, but providing patient education in a collaborative partnership is paramount to ensuring that patients and their families understand their care and what they need to do and know to stay healthy. Communicating in a way that allows patients and their families to understand what is being discussed is critical. When you speak in medical terms, use jargon or complex approaches, or provide medical information that you feel the patient should know, you are taking a medical-centered (or practitioner-centered) approach.

A typical medical-centered approach to education is to start with the disease, move on to statistics, and then go into treatment options:

Disease description

Statistics

Treatment and effectiveness

In contrast, a patient-centered approach starts with more common information (information the patient may already know), and then moves to more complex ideas. Starting with commonly understood information is a great way to help patients who might be intimidated by this new information to build confidence, as well as integrate the new information into their existing knowledge base.

General (most common) information

More specific information

The 2006 American Medical Association (AMA) report, *Improving Communication—Improving Care*, provides a more formal definition of patient-centered communication: "Patient-centered communication is respectful of and responsive to a health care user's needs, beliefs, values and preferences."[13] According to the AMA, patient-centered communication is as much about patient preferences as it is about patient safety, in addition to respecting patients' belief systems, values, and healthcare preferences.

"Reading paperwork is like emotional mountain-climbing for me. I would rather walk 10 miles than have to read, understand, and sign two forms. At least I know I can walk 10 miles."[12] This statement came from a patient who described what it's like entering the healthcare environment. Family-centered care means not only involving patients, but also providing them with the information they need in order to be involved in a way they can understand. This demonstrates the very clear link between health literacy and patient-centered care.

In addition to actually being involved in their treatment plans, patients and their families can become involved in other ways that are specific to patient education. The Joint Commission recommends in its 2006 book *Patients As Partners* that ". . . the most effective way to respond to this movement is to create and nurture patient and family advisory councils."[12] These advisory councils can provide valuable insight and feedback into patient and family education practices and materials, especially when used in a review process to ensure that your educational materials and programs are reaching the audience you intend them to reach, and that your intended messages are being received. Figure 4.7 shows an example of a feedback form that could be distributed to members of an advisory council in order to measure thoughts about patient education materials.

FIGURE 4.7 Patient and family feedback form

Our hospital would like your help in making our handouts easier to read. Please tell us what you think of this handout.

Title of handout: _____   Date: _____

Do you find this handout hard to read?   ❑ Yes   ❑ No

Does this handout contain any words that you do not understand?
                                           ❑ Yes   ❑ No
Please circle the words in the handout that you do not understand.

Does this handout answer any questions you have on the subject?
                                           ❑ Yes   ❑ No

If not, what questions do you have?

_____

_____

_____

_____

_____

Does anything on this handout hurt your feelings?   ❑ Yes   ❑ No
If yes, what?

_____

_____

_____

_____

_____

How would you change this handout to make it better or easier to understand?

_____

_____

_____

_____

_____

Patients and families are generally very eager to provide feedback on aspects of hospital care that affect them on a personal basis, such as patient education handouts. Obtaining patient and family feedback can actually help to dispel any disputes about what should or shouldn't be included in materials. For example, my facility was struggling with what template to utilize for our new, branded patient education materials. Countless meetings, debates, and discussions ensued regarding which template to use, which logo position was best, and which design was most aesthetically pleasing. I was busy tracking all the comments and feedback, analyzing them to determine which direction to take. Finally, in an "aha" moment, I decided to let patients and families choose. Rather than going through an advisory committee, I simply sat in the waiting room and asked patients which format they preferred. They overwhelmingly chose one over the other. Thus, our decision was made.

What better way to test your message than with your intended audience? Utilizing patient and family feedback is a practice that promotes involvement and helps ensure that your educational goals for patient education are met. Family-centered care and patient education have a reciprocal relationship that is interdependent for success. One cannot successfully exist without the other.

Language and Culture

The U.S. Census Bureau reported in 2004 that as the U.S. population continues to grow, so does diversity within the population. The 2005 census indicated that Hispanic-Americans total 41.3 million persons, an increase of 3.6% from the previous year, whereas the Asian population increased by 3.4%, to 14 million. Native Hawaiian, Pacific Islander, and African-American populations also increased at rates exceeding the 1% national average.[14] The concept that the United States is a "melting pot" of various cultures and ethnicities assimilated into a unitary American ethnology has become obsolete. Also, diversity within cultures exists as predominately as diversity between cultures in American society. For example, the term *Hispanic* covers many subcultures, such as Cuban, Mexican, and Argentine. As a result, there is an increased need to respond to this expansion in diversity by expanding our awareness and knowledge, and planning and providing healthcare within this new context.

Everyone is influenced by his or her culture. Whether this influence is related to how holidays are celebrated, how foods are prepared, or what world view is held, culture affects the daily life of every person. Not to be forgotten in the circle of influence are medical care and health belief systems. All cultures and different ethnic groups have beliefs related to healthcare, such as conceptualizations of health and illness, the nature of the disease, and the nature of the cause and effect.[15]

 Effectively Managing Patient Education

The culture of the United States cannot be defined by a unitary set of beliefs. Rather, society is dynamic and the effects of globalization are recasting American cultural development. America is a multiethnic and multiracial nation.[16] As a result, healthcare—in particular, patient education—has an obligation to provide information that is culturally sensitive and relevant in an ever-growing global society.

Madeleine Leininger's Culture Care Diversity and Universality Theory (1991) is a method that staff members in any setting can use to provide this type of care in a global society. The purpose or goal of the theory, according to Leininger, is "to discover and explain diverse and universal culturally based care factors influencing the health, well-being, illness, or death of individuals or groups."[17] In addition, the theory aims to provide culturally congruent care that is not only safe, but also meaningful and relevant.[17]

Essential to this purpose is an understanding of the concept of care and how it relates to culture. Leininger proposed that two elements of caring are present in every culture: an "emic" and an "etic" perspective. The emic perspective, or *generic caring*, is defined by care that is provided by a layperson and/or indigenous practices. The etic perspective, or *professional caring*, refers to nursing practices learned through formal and informal nursing education and professional nursing schools. By being aware of these different aspects of care, nurses will be able to understand how they relate to patients in terms of cultural norms.

Consistent with Leininger's theory, Sally H. Rankin and Karen Duffy Stallings in their text *Patient Education: Principles & Practice*[18] identified guidelines on how to provide patient education via a more flexible, patient-centered approach. These principles are designed to assist prenatal nurse educators in delivering individualized and culturally respectful education that may be different from the mainstream society's prenatal education program.

As an example, many minority groups in the United States are generally less-educated and of a lower income status than individuals in the dominant Caucasian culture.[19] As a result of this social status, such marginalized members of society have different needs than non-minority individuals, especially in regard to culture and language.[15] For example, many minorities have socio-cultural situations that make access to regular healthcare a challenge, so suggesting regular medical follow-up for these patients might not be the best idea. Or these patients might be low-income and unable to afford healthier food choices to manage their diabetes well, for example. Or their living conditions might predispose them to other health risks not commonly seen in higher-income patients, such as tuberculosis or lead poisoning.

Implications for patient education

Arthur Kleinman, a psychiatrist and anthropologist, is known for his work on cultural influences in healthcare. In his work, he makes a distinction between illness and disease. *Illness* is the personal experience, unique to each individual, of what is currently happening to him or her and his or her body. *Disease*, by contrast, is the healthcare professional's interpretation of what is happening in the same context. This explains why patients perceive the same diagnosis in very different ways.

Because illness is a personal perception, it's important to determine how the patient views his or her illness to provide culturally appropriate care. To reveal this perspective, Kleinman has developed the following set of eight questions, called the Kleinman Questions:[18]

- What do you call this problem?

- What do you think caused the problem?

- Why do you think it started as it did?

- What do you think the sickness does? How does it work?

- How severe is the sickness? Will it have a long or short course?

- What kind of treatment do you think the patient should receive? What are the most important results you hope he or she receives from the treatment?

- What are the chief problems the sickness has caused?

- What do you fear most about the sickness?

At times, the answers to these questions may uncover a potentially unsafe practice, such as usage of herbs or alternative therapies that may prove harmful. To address this, care providers can use the LEARN framework:[21]

- **Listen** to the patient, attempting to find out why the harmful practice is important to the patient.

- **Explain** why the practice is harmful in a biological and medical way and why the nurse is concerned about the patient's health and well-being if the practice continues. It's important to not make any disparaging remarks or otherwise offend the patient's preferred practice, but to approach the subject as objectively as possible. For example: *"Mr. Smith, I understand that you like to use nightshade as a way to combat your asthma and that you find* *it helps. I am concerned about your use of nightshade because it can interfere with your heart rate and potentially cause you to have a heart attack. Nightshade often overexcites your heart."*

- **Acknowledge** the differences but understand the shared purpose of reaching a state of health and well-being for the patient. This should be emphasized, while respectfully acknowledging each other's differences.

- **Recommend** a plan that is as mutually acceptable as possible. By acknowledging the patient's cultural norm, the nurse respects the patient's cultural needs and still alters the practice that is harmful.

- **Negotiate** the plan with the patient in a mutual relationship of partnership and involvement.

The answers to the earlier list of Kleinman Questions provide insight into how the patient views his or her condition and primary modes of treating it in his or her culture, and may reveal complementary therapies that the patient utilizes for healthcare. The responses may also provide the patient educator with an opportunity to utilize and offer complementary/alternative healing practices.

It's important to remember that there are culture-specific demographic factors in patient education, as outlined by Robert M. Huff and Michael V. Kline in their book *Promoting Health in Multicultural Populations*. These factors take into account age, gender, social class, and status, which are arguably typical demographic factors that should be considered in all patients, not just in the context of culturally appropriate care. But Huff and Kline take it a step further and identify these additional factors:

- **Literacy and education:** As discussed earlier, literacy and education levels have a significant effect on patient education and how patients are able to understand and act on information given to them. In addition, our choices of images and language may inadvertently convey the wrong concept to a patient.

- **Language:** Patients should ideally be communicated to in their primary language. Also remember that under the Culturally and Linguistically Appropriate Services standards discussed in Chapter 1, facilities are mandated to provide patients with information in their primary language to continue to receive federal funding.

- **Religious beliefs:** This goes beyond simply asking a patient whether he or she would like a visit from the hospital chaplain. It also encompasses determining how religious beliefs affect the patient's health and the patient's perspective of medicine by utilizing the Kleinman Questions listed earlier.

- **Occupation and income:** Truly assessing this in the context of providing education can assist tremendously in focusing your education endeavors to not only meet the patient's needs, but also individualize your education plan. For example, employment may place a patient at particularly high risk for accidents and exposures to health or problems. Income may give insight into the resources available to the patient once the patient is discharged from your care.

This information is critical in determining how to effectively meet patients' needs when faced with basic economic challenges. Patients facing economic challenges may have to decide each month whether they pay for their prescriptions or put food on the table, or whether they take their uninsured child to the doctor and incur an expensive office visit, or wait until it's absolutely critical and instead take the child to the emergency department. Knowing a patient's income status (or at the very least the patient's economic standing—is the patient insured?) should guide the care plan to best meet the patient's needs. A patient who does not have insurance is unlikely, for example, to go to outpatient physical therapy appointments or nutrition counseling classes. Rather, these types of patients often have to be self-reliant to maintain their health. Offering patients the option of doing therapy exercises at home, for example, or giving them easy-to-read nutrition and meal planning information, might be a more successful approach in providing patients with the information they need, rather than referring them to a potentially expensive appointment they likely will not attend.

As noted in the examples at the beginning of this chapter, health literacy, patient- and family-centered care, and language and culture are integral components to the success of any patient education endeavor, and you should consider and address them at all levels in patient education: at the bedside, in program planning, and in strategic planning. Without these pillars, patient education will not adequately support its intended audience—the patient and his or her family—and will fall short of providing any meaningful education outcomes that ultimately ensure the safety of patients.

References

1. Kirsch, I.S., Jungeblut, A., Jenkins, L., et al. *A First Look at the Results of the National Adult Literacy Survey.* Washington, DC: National Center for Education Statistics. 1993.

2. Weiss, B.D. *Health Literacy: A Manual for Clinicians.* Chicago: American Medical Association Foundation. 2003.

3. Doak, C.C., Doak, L.G., and Root, J.H. *Teaching Patients with Low Literacy Skills*, Second Edition. Philadelphia: Lippincott Williams & Wilkins, 1996.

4. The Joint Commission. *What Did the Doctor Say? Improving Health Literacy to Protect Patient Safety.* Oakbrook Terrace, IL: The Joint Commission, 2007.

5. Weiss, B.D., ed. *20 Common Problems in Primary Care.* New York City: McGraw–Hill, 1999.

6. Center for Health Care Strategies, Inc. 1997. "Health Literacy and Understanding Medical Information Fact Sheet." Available online at *www.chcs.org.* (Accessed October 6, 2008).

7. Williams, M.V., Baker, D.W., Honig, E.G., et al. "Inadequate literacy is a barrier to asthma knowledge and self care." *Chest* 114 (1998): 1008–1015.

8. Reason, J. *Human Error.* New York City: Cambridge University Press, 1990, 208.

9. Osborne, H. *Health Literacy from A to Z.* Sudbury, MA: Jones & Bartlett Publishers, Inc., 2005.

10. Ryan, J.G., Leguen, F., Weiss, B.D., et al. "Will patients agree to have their literacy skills assessed in clinical practice?" *Health Education Resources* 23(4) (2008).

11. Institute for Family-Centered Care. FAQ page. Institute for Family-Centered Care Web site, *www.familycenteredcare.org/faq.html* (accessed October 17, 2008).

12. The Joint Commission. *Patients as Partners: How to involve patients and families in their own care.* Oakbrook Terrace, IL: Joint Commission Resources, 2006.

13. AMA. "Improving Communication—Improving Care." AMA Web site, *www.mihealthandsafety.org/pdfs/06-improving-communication1.pdf* (accessed October 17, 2008).

14. America.gov. "Hispanic, Asian populations drive continued U.S. population growth." America.gov Web site, *www.america.gov/st/pubs-english/2005/October/20051005110244jmnamdeirf0.1424829.html* (accessed October 20, 2008).

15. Kleinman, A., Eisenberg, L., and Good, B. "Culture, illness and care: Clinical lessons from anthropologic and cross-cultural research." *Annals of Internal Medicine* (1978): 88.

16. Tichenor, D. 2000. "Why study the immigrant experience?" Rutgers University Web site, *http://gc2000.rutgers.edu/GC2000/MODULES/USA_IMM/default.htm* (accessed August 29, 2008).

17. Leininger, M. *Culture Care Diversity and Universality Theory*. New York City: Jones & Bartlett Publishers, Inc., 2001.

18. Rankin, S., and Duffy Stallings, K. *Patient Education: Principles & Practice*, Fourth Edition. Philadelphia: Lippincott Williams & Wilkins, 2001.

19. King, D. "Statistics". *International Journal of Childbirth Education* 15(4) (2002).

20. Glascoe, F., Oberklaid, F., Dworkin, P., et al. "Brief approaches to educating patients and parents in primary care." *Pediatrics* (1998): 101

21. Narayan, M. "Cultural Assessment and Care Planning." *Home Healthcare Nurse* 21 (2003): 611–618.

Planning for a Sustainable Future

If you were to search the Internet for the term *sustainable future*, your results would likely include several Web sites that discuss renewable energy, green practices, and environmentally friendly initiatives. Most people would not associate *patient education* with *sustainability*. Yet, the concept of sustainability is important for patient education, especially at the management level, to ensure that the processes and programs put in place can be sustained long into the future.

The idea of sustainability is really quite simple. It is based on the realization that when resources are used at a higher rate of demand than the rate at which they are supplied, the resources will be depleted. For a resource to be sustainable, the demand on the resource must be in balance with the capacity to meet the demand. As a patient education manager, you need to ensure that the changes you put in place can be sustained. You can't ask staff members to follow a new process requirement and not have the infrastructure in place to support that new requirement.

As discussed in Chapter 1, ensuring that a new process or culture shift takes hold in an organization requires that the change is anchored into the culture, and operations. If this is not the case, any change efforts you put in place risk failure as a result of the organization's inability to adapt to or sustain your change.

How Patient Education Is Organized

The patient education function within hospitals has evolved over time, as has the role of the patient education coordinator/manager. In fact, patient education as a formalized function is relatively new, with documented coordinator positions, policies, committees, and other structures beginning as recently as the late 1960s.[2] Over time, despite patient education being part of every care provider's responsibility—through job descriptions, codes of conduct, or professional practice standards—it became increasingly challenging to continue to meet the needs of patient education without some type of centralized role to help support the care staff.

Today, how patient education is organized varies widely. However, based on an original study recently released by The Advisory Board Company, centralized patient education functions usually appear to involve the development and management of patient education materials, such as hand-outs, brochures, and other organized packets of information.[3] In its study, The Advisory Board Company reviewed four hospital systems that had centralized patient education departments ranging in age from two to 10 years. All of them had at least two full-time equivalents dedicated to reviewing and developing written materials.[3]

It's interesting to learn that these organizations encountered challenges similar to those of many other patient education departments across the country. The challenges included the following:

- A lack of a formal process for distribution of written materials, ultimately leading to decreased utilization rates[3]

- An overall reduction in department staffing, resulting in longer turnaround times for patient education materials to be drafted, reviewed, and ultimately made available to the units for distribution to patients[3]

- An inability to develop (and at times) maintain patient education committees to review and approve materials, also hindering turnaround time and affecting the use of such materials at the unit level[3]

The organizations also experienced positive results, including the following:

- Furthering of a patient-/family-centered care approach through alignment of patient education materials, how patients learn best, and development of simplified care and discharge instructions[3]

- An increase in community knowledge regarding health information through the electronic availability of patient education materials[3]

- Development of patient education materials that are up to date and clinically accurate, improving the care experience[3]

Overall, the study found that centralized patient education departments focused almost exclusive-ly on the development and maintenance of patient education materials. Often, the staffing level wasn't sufficient to maintain visibility for these materials, so unit-based patient education "champions" were invested in to ensure that the materials were utilized.

It's also interesting to note that, of the centralized departments analyzed in The Advisory Board Company's recent report, not one had a mechanism in place to measure use of, and satisfaction with, the materials provided (including classes). In many cases, not only was the mechanism not in place, but metrics weren't even established. This area is often challenging, but it is a necessary component. I still struggle with determining what metrics are appropriate to demonstrate real return on investment. Something as simple as document utilization is helpful, as this can begin to tell you usage rates, but many times the true effect of patient education is the realization of better patient outcomes, such as the following:

- Fewer readmissions

- Increased patient satisfaction with patient education materials and services

- Shorter lengths of stay

- Fewer patient medication errors

Establishing that these factors are directly affected by patient education will always be a challenge; for now, correlating them and linking them appropriately will suffice for most data needs at this level.

The Advisory Board Company report also shared the following recommendations for the creation and direction of centralized patient education departments:

- **Secure physician and nurse buy-in.** This is essential. One of the bigger mistakes I made in the process of transforming how patient education is delivered at my organization was not securing physician buy-in early in the game. This led to lots of energy expenditure and meeting time trying to create buy-in after the fact, and ultimately it slowed down the project's progress. Although the project continued, it would have been more efficient if I had established physician buy-in at the beginning.

- **Implement a mechanism to gauge utilization and satisfaction rates.** Knowing how a department is performing or meeting needs (or stated goals) is crucial to understanding whether improvements are needed or additional developments are desired.

- **Ensure maximum stylistic adherence, as this improves the use and support of patient education products/materials.** Essentially, this means establishing standards for patient education materials and staying true to them so as not to dilute the brand and threaten its integrity.

- **Customize materials to specific patient populations.** This may further improve patient satisfaction. It's interesting to note that many of the departments profiled in The Advisory Board Company's report specifically did not allow customization of patient education materials; they cited fear of lack of consistency and, as a result, a decrease in overall quality.

It was interesting to read The Advisory Board Company's findings about how other centralized patient education departments function, especially because I was considering deploying a centralized patient education department in my organization. Yet, I admit to being slightly disappointed in the narrow scope that the profiled departments realized; they all worked exclusively on providing and delivering patient education materials. Although these are important tools for staff members and patients alike, patient education encompasses so much more than print materials. However, the role of most patient education managers/coordinators is to deal primarily with managing print materials and ensuring that adequate tools exist for staff members and patients.

On a daily basis, I spend most of my time reviewing and revising patient education documents to ensure that they meet readability standards. At the same time, I monitor our organization's progress related to Joint Commission accreditation and other surveys, looking for ways that patient education intersects with regulatory standards or how we can improve patient education to meet accreditation standards. My role primarily revolves around coordinating and maintaining our materials, and slowly transitioning our culture from paper-based to computer-based to make our documents easier to access and archive. See Figure 5.1 for a sample job description for a patient education coordinator.

 Effectively Managing Patient Education

FIGURE 5.1

Job description

TITLE: Patient education coordinator

DEPARTMENT: Centralized education

FUNCTIONAL PURPOSE:
Performs the primary functions of ongoing development, monitoring, maintenance, and coordination of the organizationwide patient education program.

CUSTOMER SERVICE STANDARDS:
Definition of customer: employee, visitor, physician, coworker, management, and community members
- Consistently demonstrates standards of performance
- Adheres to department-specific customer service standards

TECHNICAL SKILL CORE COMPETENCIES:
- Directs the development, implementation, promotion, distribution, and evaluation of printed, electronic, and audiovisual patient education materials
- Maintains inventory of patient education materials and resources
- Ensures the orientation of new care providers in regard to the patient education process
- Assists in other activities/special projects as assigned
- Utilizes educational databases
- Ability to format and convert documents for publishing and posting
- Utilizes MS Office programs effectively

CRITICAL THINKING CORE COMPETENCIES:
- Establishes a framework/structure for an organizationwide patient education process
- Facilitates strategic planning for the patient education process
- Identifies patient education needs through data collection and analysis
- Participates in interdepartmental activities, including interpretation of policies and procedures as necessary to facilitate and optimize patient care
- Participates in quality improvement and Joint Commission–related activities and provides input on quality indicators and standards
- Possesses expertise in the continuum of clinical care
- Utilizes project management skills
- Demonstrates performance improvement skills

FIGURE 5.1 # Job description (cont.)

- Incorporates knowledge of adult learning principles in the development of patient education materials
- Shows ability to assess the educational needs of patients related to learning style preference, age, barriers to learning and cultural needs
- Possesses excellent organizational and prioritization skills

INTERPERSONAL CORE COMPETENCIES:
- Clarifies roles and responsibilities and ensures interdisciplinary involvement in patient education
- Collaborates with dedicated resources within product lines to meet identified patient needs
- Acts as a resource or consultant to individuals, groups, and departments organizationwide and seeks consultation with outside experts to achieve patient education goals
- Exhibits strong change management skills
- Demonstrates effective meeting facilitation skills
- Possesses ability to negotiate with vendors

DEPARTMENT-SPECIFIC:
- Participates as active and respectful member of the work group
- Provides open, honest, constructive feedback to members of the team
- Demonstrates a willingness to assist other department members
- Effectively utilizes appropriate hardware/software necessary to perform the role
- Contributes to the successful achievement of department goals and objectives
- Initiates opportunities for improvement in role, department, and processes utilizing Plan-Do-Check-Act
- Utilizes human and material resources in a cost-effective manner and within budget guidelines
- Acts accountably for appropriate intake and intradepartmental referrals and handoffs
- Abides by department policy and procedures
- Delivers culturally sensitive services

ORGANIZATIONAL REQUIREMENTS:
- Adheres to organizational practices relating to confidentiality
- Complies with organizational training requirements on life safety matters (emergency codes, MSDS, etc.) and standard precautions

 Effectively Managing Patient Education

FIGURE 5.1	Job description (cont.)

- Abides by organizational policies and procedures
- Maintains confidential information by discussing private and/or sensitive matters only with the appropriate persons and only in appropriate locations

EDUCATION, LICENSURE/CERTIFICATION, AND EXPERIENCE:
- Master's degree preferred.
- Five years of experience in clinical nursing. BSN required.
- Current nursing licensure in [insert state].
- Past experience with patient education processes preferred.

ORGANIZATIONAL REPORTING RELATIONSHIP:
- Reports to the Director of Education.

AMERICANS WITH DISABILITIES ACT (ADA) ESSENTIAL ELEMENTS:
- Ability to effectively communicate with employees and visitors verbally and in writing
- Analytical ability to resolve problems that require the use of basic scientific, mathematical, or technical principles

ADA QUALIFICATIONS:
- Ability to write and speak
- Able to hear with or without accommodation
- Work requires lifting and/or carrying objects weighing up to 25 pounds
- Work requires the ability to reach and grasp objects
- Work requires manual dexterity
- Work requires the ability to enter words and data into a computer or similar device

As noted earlier, patient education can take many forms beyond print materials, including patient and family resource centers. This is a new approach to offering health information in a library-type setting where patients, their families, and the community can research issues while obtaining basic health coaching from a health educator. Similar to resource centers are patient and family skills labs, where family members who have to take care of their loved ones at home can learn how to perform essential tasks in a controlled lab setting. This allows caregivers to become familiar with injections, dressing changes, total parenteral nutrition (intravenous) feedings, and other skills they will have to perform at home.

These are just two examples of additional forms of patient education. It also involves the integration of community education and outreach, intersection with marketing, and much more. This chapter will equip you to plan for the future of your facility's patient education program by taking all of these issues into account.

Advocating for Resources

As a patient education manager, it is your job to make healthcare leaders aware of what a patient education program requires to succeed, as well as to advocate for resources to ensure that patient education needs are met. A common mistake is to assume that once leaders are aware of the role of patient education and its effect on patient care, patient safety, strategic goals, and satisfaction scores, they will automatically provide resources (in terms of both funding and staffing) to take things to the next level. Rather, the patient education manager must be the one to continuously and effectively advocate for necessary resources and demonstrate probable outcomes attainable *with* those resources. An effective way to advocate for those resources is to develop a business case.

Developing a business case and defining outcomes

A business case is similar in concept to solving a problem that you have identified. For example, the problem may be a lack of resources (such as staff members, budget dollars, or processes) to adequately and efficiently support a new initiative. Suppose you succeed in initiating a process for approval of patient education materials, but as a result, a massive influx of materials is coming your way, and you cannot approve them for patient use in a timely manner. If this continues, users may start to circumvent the system because they are dissatisfied. The business case then attempts to answer the "What if?" question: What happens if this particular course of action is taken or not taken?

Asking this question and thinking it through can assist you in furthering patient education in your facility. Knowing how and when to use a business case helps the patient education manager go beyond the basics.

The process for developing a solid business case typically comprises the following steps:[1]

1. **Define the opportunity.** Describe the problem in detail and identify the objectives your business case will address. For example, the problem may be that your organization lacks a centralized method for approving and disseminating patient education materials that are standardized, and as a result, the information given to patients varies widely, which often results in confusion and dissatisfaction. In addition, patient safety is at risk because there isn't a way to centrally verify that the information given out is current and evidence-based.

2. **Identify alternatives.** To demonstrate that you have thought through the situation carefully, identify several solutions to your situation and then analyze three in depth. With the example in Step 1, you have a few alternatives:

   - Do nothing

   - Acquire all of the self-authored materials from the staff, catalog them, and centralize them

   - Throw them all out and hire a vendor to write them instead

3. **Gather data and choose a time frame.** Obtain information on each alternative and estimate how long each alternative will take to implement. So, if hiring a vendor is an alternative, obtain a proposal and cost estimate from the vendor and further analyze the pros and cons based on the results. Do the same with the other options. Would the unit managers be willing to have their key staff members spend their time rewriting materials to meet new standards and centralizing them in one catalog? How much time do you think that would take? This may involve drafting a preliminary timeline.

4. **Choose an alternative and assess risks.** Choose and identify your recommendation based on your analysis and data. Be sure to include how you will approach any risk associated with your recommendation. A great way to perform a risk assessment is to conduct a SWOT (strengths, weaknesses, opportunities, threats) analysis; more on this shortly.

5. **Create a high-level implementation plan.** Demonstrate at a high level what outcomes you expect to achieve if your proposal is accepted. Often, this is presented as a work plan. If you chose to hire a vendor, you need to determine what must occur to make that

happen. You will need funding, as well as assistance from your information technology department, as the vendor integrates with your existing infrastructure.

6. **Communicate your case.** Compile all your information into a document and present it to decision-makers within your organization. This generally begins with sending your written report to a few key leaders who you think may need to see this document, particularly your reporting director. Your director needs to be one of the first people to see what you have proposed so that he or she will not be surprised by any conversations that may circulate regarding the proposal. In addition, it's good to remember that, although you are drafting the proposal, ultimately the accountability for ensuring that it happens (if it's approved) from a resource standpoint *is* your reporting director. He or she also can help advocate for you when it's time to sell your proposal to key decision-makers in the organization.

It's also important to identify how your organization handles business cases, as some organizations may have particular templates and formats. This is a good item to investigate before you dive in too deep. I began my research for a business plan on the Internet, and I looked at several examples before developing my plan. Ultimately, that was a great way to initiate discussing my plan with my director and my mentor, but in reality, I had to change my format a bit to accommodate my organization's expectations. At that time, I also found out who my audience was, which helped me to reframe my content slightly. My audience was going to be primarily vice presidents, so I had to provide more background/historical information, as they were likely not as entrenched in the content as me or my reporting director. Appendix 1 provides an example of a business case, and Appendix 2 provides an example of a work plan.

The Art of Persuasion

Now that you have created a business case, you need to sell it to the decision-makers in your organization and be persuasive in your sell. But what does it mean to be persuasive? You need to be able to sway viewpoints, be influential and capture attention, and cause others to reconsider their prior opinions and join forces with you to support your cause. Persuasion is defined as "a process that enables you to change or reinforce others' attitudes, opinions or behaviors."[1] This process can vary in length and intensity; it can occur in one meeting or over the course of several years and several discussions. It requires a blend of skills that call for diligent data collection and analysis, as well as superb communication skills, all while appealing to your audience's emotions.

 Effectively Managing Patient Education

Persuasion is an important skill for patient education managers to have, as it will assist you in your endeavors to grow patient education within your organization. As mentioned earlier in this book, patient education managers need to constantly sell and advocate for resources, as well as demonstrate the value of patient education. Many times, you can accomplish these tasks through the powers of persuasion. The reality is that many priorities compete within healthcare, and all of them have merit and require resources that are hard to secure. Being able to secure those scare resources requires being persuasive.

In fact, persuasion is useful in many situations, from advocating for a pay raise to selling a product. In a position such as patient education manager, where there are often no direct reports, persuasion is crucial to ensure that others accomplish any patient education–related goals. Persuasion became particularly critical in my role when I needed several staff nurses and clinicians to champion the review of thousands of patient education handouts and rewrite them to meet readability standards that I had set. Although in theory, many staff members could agree that our patient education materials and how our organization handled them needed to be fixed, committing to the real work was a challenge. In many cases, managers submitted cost estimates for their staff members' time (often in the thousands of dollars) to commit to this endeavor; was my department going to pay for that? I kept the critical areas in mind as I made my arguments and was able to secure a solid group of staff members who were committed to transforming our patient education materials.

Given that persuasion is a process, it's important to recognize the critical areas around which all persuasive dialogue must revolve:[1]

- **Credibility:** Acquire expertise while simultaneously building trusting relationships

- **Common ground:** All goals are framed on this "common ground" viewpoint and how goals share common values

- **Supporting information:** Reinforce your position with storytelling and data

- **Deep understanding of emotion:** Be able to connect with the audience on an emotional level

People generally respond to persuasion in one of two ways: consciously or subconsciously. Consciously, they may have actively thought about your proposal, analyzed your findings, and come to a logical conclusion and subsequent acceptance of your recommendations. Or subconsciously, they may make their decisions based on "gut reactions" that may have nothing to do with any facts or findings.

Often these types of subconscious decisions are based simply on relationships. Think about how many times you may have rejected an idea that had merit because the idea came from someone you didn't respect. This is why relationship-building is extremely important in the patient education role, and why visibility and networking at the leadership level are critical to success.

Several times, I have attempted to persuade a leader to support one of my recommendations, but because we did not have an established relationship, the leader was quick to reject my ideas. After I was allowed to integrate with leadership more frequently (at various leadership meetings, retreats, and other development opportunities), the situation improved, and I found it much easier to garner support. I formed an established relationship and a level of trust with leadership. That can happen only when you're allowed to interact with leaders outside of asking them for support or persuading them to do something.

The Patient Education Manager's Toolbox

A good patient education manager will have a few tricks up his or her sleeve to help get the message across to all members of the staff. The following techniques will prove to be useful when persuading different staff members of the importance of patient education.

Kick-start your ideas: CAP tools

Thinking about patient education and all of its possibilities can easily overwhelm you. How do you ensure that all areas are examined, and all possibilities and contingencies are considered? The change acceleration process (CAP) tools[2] can assist. These tools are designed to teach you how to help staff members adapt to and accept new processes and methodologies. The CAP process involves the following steps:[2]

1. **Create a shared need.** This entails getting individuals on board with the reason change is required, through data, demonstration, demand, or diagnosis. Essentially, the need for change must be greater than the urge to resist the change. Most important is highlighting any dissatisfaction with the status quo.

2. **Shape a vision.** This is where you clearly define a scope of change that everyone can understand.

3. **Mobilize commitment.** In this critical step, you identify the key stakeholders, analyze any predicted resistance, and plan how to gain strong commitment for your endeavor by mobilizing people to invest in your proposed change.

4. **Make change last.** Once a new process or change is in place, you must plan for and reinforce the change throughout the organization. Most efforts will fail if the change is not at least 50% sustainable.[1] We tend to spend most of our energy and time *launching* a new initiative rather than determining how it will be sustained and institutionalized over time.[1]

5. **Monitor progress.** Set your benchmarks and success measures so that you know when you've got it right.

Utilizing CAP tools is a great way to kick-start your ideas, especially improvement projects. Often, expanding patient education services can be viewed as an improvement project. Think about your current role. If it comprises merely creating and distributing materials, you know from reading this book that numerous other aspects of patient education are just as important to consider and address. Patient education can mean comprehensive health literacy programs, a patient and family consumer health library, community education classes, a patient and family skills lab, research and data collection, and more. All those functions require tangible things such as money and staffing, but how do you know how many staff members you need and what the scope of each function should be? The CAP tools can help you answer these questions.

Create a shared need: SWOT analysis

A SWOT analysis is a fairly common tool and is a great way to demonstrate why an improvement or change needs to occur. As noted earlier, SWOT stands for *strengths, weaknesses, opportunities,* and *threats.* SWOT analysis allows you to position your proposed change in both positive and negative contexts while demonstrating that the proposal for change was analyzed. Figure 5.2 shows an example of a SWOT analysis about building a case for self-authoring versus hiring a vendor to write patient education materials.

FIGURE 5.2	SWOT analysis for writing patient education materials versus hiring a vendor

Strengths	**Weaknesses**
Organizational willingness to align	Consistency
Executive support	Organizational standards
Many frontline staff members invested in writing materials	Budget dollars
	Archiving
Homegrown documents; allows for distinct customization	Community image
Opportunities	**Threats**
Linkage to *Hospital Consumer Assessment of Healthcare Providers and Systems*; trending in qualitative patient perception of care	Regulatory bodies
	Competition most likely will penetrate hospital service area
Linkage to patient-/family-centered care approach at The Office of Minority Health	Patient safety
	Litigation
	Patient perception

Shape your vision: More of/less of exercise

The "more of/less of" exercise helps you to spell out your vision in identifiable and behavior-based terms. It also will reveal what will happen if your proposal or improvement comes to fruition. With this tool, you spend time brainstorming what you'd like to see more of and less of in the future.

For example, in an expanded, integrated patient education services department, you might want to see more of a focus on staff development classes highlighting patient education, a patient library, and a well-staffed skills lab. At the same time, you may wish to see less of a focus on patient education materials, less time spent duplicating work that was started but not finished due to lack of a coordinated approach, and less dissatisfaction from nursing leaders who are looking for measurable results that you can't provide because of limited resources. This exercise is great to conduct in a group setting, but it's also useful on your own when you're attempting to gather your thoughts.

 Effectively Managing Patient Education

Mobilize commitment: Action planning

Action planning is an absolute must at the conclusion of almost any meeting where real work needs to be done and decisions are made. Once your team members have been identified, mapping out a WWW (who, what, when) action plan is a great way to ensure that the group stays committed to the process. See Figure 5.3 for a sample action plan.

FIGURE 5.3   Action plan: Deciding who, what, and when

Who	What	When
Rebecca	Develop a process for auditing the current patient education materials	2 weeks
Bill	Design a database to catalog the inventory of materials	3 weeks

Make change last: Force field analysis

Also called "help or hinder," force field analysis helps you to assess what types of resistance or support you may encounter for your initiative. Understanding this will help you to build action plans around people who are hindering the process and build upon those people who are allies. See Figure 5.4 for an example of the force field analysis tool, as well as directions on how to use it.

FIGURE 5.4　　　　Force field analysis tool

That help/hinder figure, or Force field analysis tool, is a form that you could use in a meeting (on an easel or whiteboard, for example) to help brainstorm factors that either help or "hinder" a specific initiative. In my organization, we use the tool by drawing it on an easel, using Post-It notes to have people write down an idea or concept, and placing those ideas in either the "help" or "hinder" side. It's a nice visual to facilitate discussion and keep things moving.

Example of how to use:

Scenario: You are facilitating a discussion to determine next steps in opening up a patient and family resource center, a unique place within your hospital that would provide a destination for patients and families to come and learn more about health-related topics, browse books and journals, speak with a health educator, and/or practice new skills such as subcutaneous injections. During your discussion, you suggest it might be a good idea to explore and identify what would both help and hinder your project, so you decide to use the force field analysis. Doing so will allow you to:

1. Leverage those things that are a help to strengthen your project
2. Develop action plans to proactively subvert those that may hinder your progress

Help:	Hinder:
• Community desire • Potential alignment with strategic vision • New construction plans still being approved • Potential to collaborate with existing medical library	• Lack of funding • Physicians want own library space away from patients

　　　　　　Effectively Managing Patient Education

Force field analysis, along with the tools and techniques mentioned in the preceding sections, is a tool you can use to build for your future. Although you can use these tools and techniques for any project, large or small, all of them provide an excellent framework for establishing what you'd like to see, in clear, measurable terms, for an integrated, comprehensive patient education department. They allow you to take patient education to the next level.

Key Takeaways for the New Patient Education Manager

If you are new to the role of patient education manager, here are some principles by which to lead your working life.

Take time to educate yourself

When I began my role in patient education, the role was new for both me and my organization. I always had a passion for education, particularly educating patients, so the role was a natural fit for me. At the time, I think the organization was aware that patient education at the system level needed some care and attention, but leaders weren't sure what that entailed or what it meant. That small bit of ambiguity and uncertainty was okay, because I believed that's what the organization wanted *me* to define.

I entered the role with what I now know was a superficial understanding of patient education. My background as a labor and delivery staff nurse told me that patient education was important. I knew patients needed to be educated; I also knew my patients who were first-time parents needed *lots* of education. And as an RN, I had a lot of information to share. As a staff development nurse, I knew adult education principles and figured the same approach for patients was required. I also knew that health literacy was a major concern, but I did not understand much regarding the details.

Going into the role, I had the advantage of a director who knew patient education was broken, for lack of a better word, at our organization, and she allowed me the freedom and flexibility to take the time I needed to just sit and think about its current state, what needed to be done, and how to do it. That was when I started researching the practices and principles of patient education. Without this time to fully educate myself—not only on current practices, but also on the current state of my organization—I wouldn't have been well-equipped to present a case for change and engage the organization in what would become a long journey toward transformation.

Make your recommendations

Once I had a more solid understanding of patient education and could see where our gaps existed, I began to make my presence and my opinion known. I started that process carefully and nonconfrontationally, because not only was I a new employee, but I was also not a titled leader, and thus had to earn my authority and credibility. That may have been one of the greatest struggles in my new career, and is why I believe and advocate that any patient education position, at the system or corporate level, needs to be held by a titled leader. This will not solve every problem you encounter, but it will shorten the length of time you'll need to overcome some of the eventual barriers.

Making my recommendations known was a two-part lesson. First, I learned how to make my recommendations succinct and sound, so as to not cause confusion or angst and to get straight to the point of what I was asking the organization to do. Second, I learned that how I presented my recommendations was largely dependent on my skills and what type of leader I was. My biggest regret is that, although I thoroughly analyzed the organization's state regarding patient education, I neglected to adequately assess the key players in the organization, which resulted in my inadvertently making some political missteps. They were easily corrected, but were not something I wanted to do during my first six months in a new role.

By communicating my recommendations at the leadership level, I accomplished three important goals: I gained visibility in the organization, I gained credibility as an expert, and I was able to set expectations and goals for the organization. In fact, I believe that communicating across the organization enabled me to gain support and mobilize a large team of patient care staff members to make a three-year investment in transforming patient education. Communicating my recommendations led me to form a positive and productive relationship with a senior-level executive who supported my initiative, provided valuable insight and experience, removed barriers, and provided one-on-one mentoring to me and helped me to grow as a professional and eventual leader. That relationship proved to be one of the most valuable factors that helped to transform patient education at my organization, and I can't stress that enough. When patient education has the interest and attention of senior leaders, the chances are high that change can take place and positive things can happen, ultimately resulting in quality patient care and improved patient safety.

Be persistent

If patient education is your passion, as it is mine, persistence is fairly easy to come by, because you won't rest until you meet your goals for an ideal patient education system. But admittedly, persistence takes energy, and often it's easy to think that perhaps you're in the wrong organization; you begin to question whether the organization is ready to make the necessary changes and investments it says it wants to make. But really, you're facing what everyone else is facing: competing priorities. This is why being able to talk the talk of leadership, being persuasive in your positions and opinions, and coming equipped with data to support your cause can help you to strengthen your position, which eventually will pay off with additional resources and energy devoted to ensuring that patient education is brought to the required level.

I hope this book will be a great starting point for you as a patient education manager—particularly if you're new to your role or are wondering how you can transform how patient education is delivered in your organization. I trust that the tools and techniques you've read about on these pages will help you to achieve your goals.

References

1. "Harvard ManageMentor PLUS—Creating a Business Case." *http://harvardbusinessonline.hbsp.harvard.edu/ b02/en/elearning/elearning_hmm.jhtml.* (Accessed October 14, 2008).

2. Giloth, B.E. "Management of patient education in U.S. hospitals: Evolution of a concept." *Patient Education and Counseling* 15 (1990): 101–111.

3. The Advisory Board Company. July 2007. "Structure and Operations of Centralized Education Departments in Health Systems." Original Inquiry Brief. *www.advisoryboardcompany.com.*

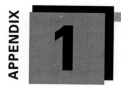

Proposal for the Creation of Patient and Family Education Services

Need/Problem Statement

Community Hospital has followed a decentralized process for patient education for some time, and in 2005, it established the need for a centralized approach via the creation of a patient education coordinator position. Since that time, the demand for patient and health education services has increased, and an even more structured, coordinated, and supportive approach must evolve to meet the needs of the enterprise.

Goal

Establish and implement a system-level department that is responsible for patient education program development and support across the enterprise.

Objective

Implement a patient and family education services function within the education department, with the creation of a full-time *patient and family education services manager* and a full-time *health education specialist.*

Historical Perspective

With a decentralized approach, Community Hospital units, departments, and clinics had virtually no patient education support, and would often use valuable clinician time to write patient education materials, purchase materials, or develop patient education programs. As a result, no coordinated patient education program exists.

Current State

Community Hospital is restructuring how patient education materials are developed, distributed, and stored, and has implemented specific standards and guidelines for patient materials. Currently, newly developed patient education materials are managed solely by the patient education coordinator, who meets with the authors and assists in planning, developing, writing/editing, and formatting, as well as selecting graphics. Community Hospital has an inventory of 11,967 patient education documents and develops on average one to two pieces of new material each week. Turnaround times for patient education services are around six to eight weeks, which is not meeting the organization's needs. Current patient education services include:

- Review of existing materials for suitability to patients
- Development of educational objectives for patient education pieces
- Editing and reformatting of patient education documents
- Design/word placement
- Graphics selection or obtainment
- Facilitation of patient review of final piece

A more proactive approach to managing patient education material development is necessary to provide timely service to the enterprise.

In addition, the current patient and family resource center is unmanaged and unstaffed, leaving a huge gap in service to patients and the community and a large loss of potential for expansion of those services, such as through a patient and family skills lab, outpatient wellness classes, and retail services.

In summary, the current state does not allow for the following:

- Expansion of patient and family education programs
- Growth of patient and family education and full integration into the fabric of Community Hospital
- Research and data collection

Structure and Services

Community Hospital Patient and Family Education Services will operate under three service lines: **planning and development, support,** and **community outreach.** The following services will be provided; these services are either not provided currently or are provided only minimally:

Planning and development

- Assessment and evaluation of hospital needs for patient and family education

- Planning, implementation, and evaluation of health education programs, including defining measurable program objectives that are consistent with strategic goals

- Planning, implementation, and evaluation of a health literacy program to formally address the recommendations by The Joint Commission and the Institute for Healthcare Improvement

Support

- One-on-one support to departments/clinicians (subject matter experts) in development of patient education pieces, ensuring that standards are met and the pieces are fulfilling an identified need

- Standards for bedside practice, including accreditation standards support

- Maintenance of a patient education catalog, including developing processes regarding material reviews, updates, and archival

- Support and alignment of community education efforts across service lines

- Consultative services for patient education best practices

- Continuing education for staff members on patient education skills

Community outreach

- Assessment of community needs for health education

- Formal management of the patient and family resource center and expansion of its services, as well as expansion of the patient education concept to additional facilities

- Establishment of processes that facilitate patient/community member input on patient education programs and materials

A draft Work Plan is attached, outlining first steps and priorities if this proposal is accepted.

Organizational chart

The following is a proposed organizational chart for Community Hospital Patient and Family Education Services within the education department:

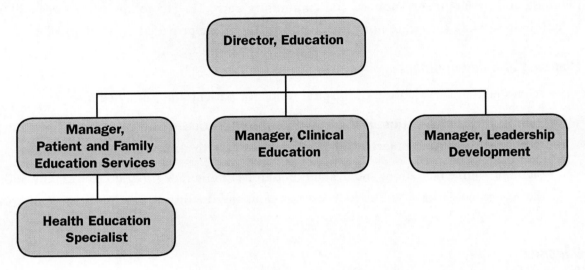

Alignment with Strategic Goals

Development of this function within the education department aligns with two strategic goals for Community Hospital:

Patient-centered care

Creating a structured, staffed department function devoted to patient and family education allows Community Hospital to fully integrate patient-/family-centered care into a critical aspect of healthcare. Without this growth of patient and family education, support of this strategic goal will be severely limited.

Quality

Expansion of patient and family education allows for potential quality improvement and a more productive, seamless approach to a critical patient service.

 Effectively Managing Patient Education

Benchmarking

The Joint Commission has stated, relative to formal patient education departments, that:

Patient and family education is an integral part of high quality patient care. Those organizations that provide targeted, comprehensive and appropriate education to their patients and families encourage patient participation, which can improve health outcomes, shorten lengths of stay and save money for a facility. In fact, it has been said that for every dollar spent on patient education, three to four dollars are saved.

—The Joint Commission Guide to Patient & Family Education, 2003

A review of other organizations' patient education structures indicated wide variations, from having a single person responsible for patient education to having elaborate departments with several supporting functions. A common theme was that the more developed and comprehensive the department, the more services could be provided, which resulted in better outcomes.

A competing hospital has a patient education department consisting of a manager, several educators, and program assistants. As a result of sufficient budget dollars and human resources, this patient education department was able to expand its services to include a patient resource center, which recently added a patient and family skills lab. This resource center has allowed patients and their families to learn self-care skills with the help of a qualified health educator before being discharged to home, which has resulted in improved health outcomes for the hospital's patients.

Unfortunately, limited data is available on patient education outcomes and structures. The most recent data on hospitalwide management structures for patient education suggested the following:

Does the existence of hospital wide management structures, such as the presence of a Patient Education Manager and supporting personnel, make a difference in terms of the patient education provided? Limited data suggest they do.

—Managing Hospital-Based Patient Education, 1993

Timeline

The creation of Patient and Family Education Services and the subsequent hiring of a full-time health education specialist would commence immediately upon approval of this endeavor. Support is needed urgently during this critical time when Community Hospital is in the midst of centralizing patient education and risks putting into place a system that we cannot support.

Budget Implications

- Current salary for patient education coordinator: $35.45/hour. **Net increase of dollars needed to bump to manager pay grade.**

- Current salary for education program planner: $22.30/hour. **Net increase of dollars needed to bump to higher pay range consistent with the market value of a health education specialist.**

- Replacement for education program planner (1.0 full-time equivalent at $16.31–$24.47) *or* transitioning that function to an existing education partner.

Next Steps

- Approval of the creation of Patient and Family Education Services by the management committee

- Development of a job description for the manager of Patient and Family Education Services

- Development of a health education specialist job description

- Transition planning

Risks

Without a formalized structure in place to support enterprise patient education, Community Hospital risks the following:

- Investing resources into centralizing patient education print materials, but lacking the infrastructure to continue its support and assist its growth in line with the rest of the organization

- Limited quality of patient education as a whole, negatively affecting health outcomes of our patients and families and potentially resulting in untimely readmissions and complications

- An atrophic patient and family resource center not operating at its potential, with virtually no room for concept expansion to the rest of the enterprise

- Integration and identity issues with recently acquired clinic practice patient education

With the growth of Community Hospital, it is only fitting that a vital patient service such as patient education grows as well.

2

Patient and Family Education Services Sample Work Plan

Patient Education Mission Statement

Community Hospital supports patients, their families, and the community in their quest for health information and knowledge by providing quality health education that is informative and individualized.

	Tactics	When	Comments
Planning and development	Explore methods for data collection on patient and family education needs for Community Hospital Explore and develop services for patient/family resource center; prepare for expansion Explore and recommend strategies for wide-scale translation efforts for patient education materials Create a preliminary plan for health literacy program	Within first 12 months	As defined by the Partnerships for Patients Work Plan

	Tactics	When	Comments
Support	Create and implement a process for patient education material support via one-on-one consultation with the health educator and subject matter expert	Immediately upon hire of health educator	These functions are critical to the success of the Patient Education Solution Project (centralizing of patient education)
	Create and formalize communication and process venues for patient education news, best practices, and recognition awards	Immediately upon hire of health educator	
	Analyze and define tools needed to ensure long-term success of the Patient Education Solution Project		
Community outreach	Evaluate current methods for community input on programming and determine methods of expansion and formalization	Within first 10–12 months	
	Explore a potential alliance with Community Education		

Culture of Patient Safety Toolkit: Activities for Use at Department Meetings

The following toolkit was created by my organization to teach our staff members about creating and working in a culture of safety. The toolkit has been generalized so that any facility could follow the general principles while modifying the material as needed. It was created so that any manager within our hospital would be able to pick up this toolkit and, without much instruction, be able to facilitate an activity or discussion around the listed topics at unit meetings. Use the objectives and prompt questions to discuss your organization's culture of safety.

Feedback and Communication

Evaluate the extent to which staff members are informed about errors that occur, are given feedback regarding changes implemented, and if they discuss ways to prevent errors.

Activity—Improving organizational performance

Objective: Explore with staff members their relationships to publicly reported data about the organization.

Directions:

1. Ask staff members the following questions:

    • What data is publicly reported on our organization?

    • What does publicly reported data look like for our organization?

2. Explain to the staff how to access publicly reported data from The Joint Commission:

   • Go to *www.qualitycheck.org*.

   • Choose the state and city in which your organization is located via the drop-down menus on the right-hand side of the screen. Then click the Search button.

   • In the Type of Provider/Certification pull-down menu, select Hospitals and then click the Search button.

   • Scroll through the results. When you find your hospital, click the View Accreditation Quality Report link.

   • Click the See Detail link next to the National Patient Safety Goal report in which you are interested.

3. Explain to the staff how to access publicly reported data from The LeapFrog Group:

   • Go to *www.leapfroggroup.org*.

   • Click For Consumers.

   • Select "Click here to find Leapfrog Hospital Ratings".

   • Enter the city and state location of your facility, and click Compare Now.

   • Review the resultant data.

   • Select the Click to Change Treatment drop-down menu on the left-hand side of the screen, choose the High Risk Delivery checkbox, and view the resultant data.

4. Explain to the staff how to access publicly reported data from the Centers for Medicare & Medicaid Services (CMS):

   • Go to *www.hospitalcompare.hhs.gov*.

   • Note that:

     – The Hospital Compare tool is "a quality tool for adults, including people with Medicare." Hospitals can vary in the quality of care they provide. This Web site was created to help consumers see how well the hospitals in their area care for their patients and to compare the quality of care hospitals provide. As of June 2007, CMS increased the number of quality measures, reporting 22 process measures and two outcome measures. Patient satisfaction measures were added in early 2008 to provide even more detail to help make available the information consumers need for healthcare decision-making.

- The Hospital Compare tool allows consumers to see the recommended care that an adult should receive if being treated for a heart attack, heart failure, or pneumonia or if having surgery.

- The quality of care information comes from hospitals that submit their data voluntarily from their patient records. The information is converted to rates that measure how well the hospitals care for their patients. In addition to reporting quality measures, Hospital Compare includes tools consumers can use to start a conversation with their physician or hospital about what the information means and how they can best get the care they need.

- Click the Find and Compare Hospitals button.

- Choose an option and enter your search criteria. Then click the Continue button.

- Choose a search option and then click Continue.

- Choose which hospital you want to compare to your own, and click the Compare button.

Frequency of Events Reported

Mistakes of the following types are reported within our facility:

- Mistakes caught and corrected before affecting the patient (near miss)

- Mistakes with no potential to harm the patient

- Mistakes that could harm the patient but that do not

Activity—Incident reporting process

Objective: Reeducate the staff on the incident reporting process.

Directions: Using each of the scenarios below, discuss what your hospital's reporting process is and how a staff member should have handled each incident.

Patient injury scenario

Patient: Iva Soreleg

Identification #: 000001

Iva was scheduled to receive a dose of Coumadin 5 mg PO at 1800. Dr. Van Nostrom had ordered a PT/INR be done the morning of October 31. Dawn Tired, the day-shift RN, called the PT/INR results to the MD (results: PT 28 INR 2.6) at 1430 and received an order to hold the Coumadin at 1800 today only. Dawn, the PM nurse forgot to tell you, about the new order. You appreciate the patient care reports and use them daily. Unfortunately, the report you were referring to for Iva's plan of care had been printed before the new order was processed. You gave the Coumadin, and discovered the error when you went to chart it. You called Dr. Van Nostrom, who told you to hold the Coumadin until further notice and repeat the PT/INR in the morning.

Employee injury scenario

Patient: Al Coholic

Identification #: 000002

On Monday, December 7, you an RN, are assigned to care for Mr. Coholic, who is going through alcohol withdrawal. He is somewhat confused, can be combative, and is unsteady on his feet. His doctor has ordered that he can be up with assistance only. He is on fall precautions and has a bed check. When you enter his room at 1400 to take his vital signs, you find him on the floor. He is asking you to help him up and is complaining that his left hip is hurting. You call for help. The nurse comes in and assesses the patient, and both of you help him back to bed. As you are assisting with this task, you experience pain shooting down your left leg. You call the emergency room, and they ask that you come down to be assessed. The emergency room doctor advises you to go home and call Employee Health in the morning.

Environmental safety scenario

Location: Hospital grounds

You are coming to work on November 12, and as you are walking across the parking lot, you slip and fall on a patch of ice. You do not immediately notice an injury and proceed to work. As soon as you get into the building, you notify maintenance about the ice in the parking lot.

Handoffs

Important patient care information is transferred across hospital units and during shift changes.

Objective: Demonstrate handoffs for direct and indirect patient care.

Directions:

1.   Prior to performing the activity with the staff, the facilitator (manager) reviews the following grid.

2.   Print out the grid and cut into two sets of slips, one describing situations and the other describing handoffs.

3.   Give staff members the papers and have them match the situation to the handoff.

Situation	Handoff
You have a 23-hour-observation patient. The physician just wrote an order to keep the patient for another day. What do you do?	Call admitting and have your patient's status changed from observation to inpatient.
Your patient is on schedule for a total hip replacement, and you notice the patient's potassium is 3.0. What do you do?	Call the anesthesiologist who will be caring for the patient.
You observe water leaking from the ceiling tiles on your unit. Who do you notify?	Call facilities, or if after hours, call the operator and ask that the facilities staff member on call be paged.
You have a blood pressure cuff that needs to be replaced. Who do you notify?	Go to the intranet, submit a form, and notify your manager.
Your computer workstation locked up. Who do you call?	Call the information services department.
Your glucometer is not downloading properly into the computer system. Who do you call?	Call the laboratory point of care.

Situation	Handoff
You pick up a hamper full of linen and feel a "twinge" in your back. What do you do?	Fill out a Safety Incident Report and an Accident Investigation Form, both available through Employee Health. Then notify your manager and Employee Health.
You receive a needlestick. What do you do?	Squeeze the area to express blood from the wound. Then wash the area vigorously with soap and water. Go to the emergency room for an evaluation. Then fill out a Safety Incident Report. Notify your manager and Employee Health.
You identify that there are never enough thermometers in the department to service patients. What do you do?	Notify your manager in writing of the request, the rationale for the request, and the number of thermometers currently in the department.

  Effectively Managing Patient Education

Q&A with Susan Kanack

Q Can you describe your responsibilities on a daily basis?

A My responsibilities on a daily basis include, at the operational level: writing, editing and revising patient education materials to ensure that they meet standards for account readability and patient-centeredness; conducting periodic chart audits to determine how patient education is being documented and to identify areas of concern and areas for improvement/targeted education; developing educational offerings for staff members about best practice patient education practice, such as documentation and writing effective handouts; and consulting with various providers in the organization on health literacy issues. At the strategic level: attending meetings and developing action plans/tactics related to organizational goals, ensuring patient education is considered and represented; leading patient education steering committee meetings; and leading system integration meetings for patient education practices/processes as our organization grows and begins to acquire other healthcare systems. In addition, encouraging community involvement both at the state and local levels in health literacy initiatives helps to strengthen our image to the community, as well as be on the forefront of solution development for such a large health problem (health literacy).

Q How do you teach your staff about providing patient education?

A Teaching staff members, especially in the acute care setting, is always a challenge. Staff time away from patient care duties is a premium; combined with high acuity levels and short staffing, this makes reaching out and educating staff a challenge. My organization utilizes a learning management system (LMS) to track and deliver staff education. Computer-based learning modules (CBL) are great ways to develop course content/curriculum that staff members can access on their "down time" when it is convenient for them, as opposed to having them attend an instructor-led class that takes them away from the unit. I utilize CBLs to deliver education that I feel is primarily review material or fundamentals—mostly theory components and information sharing about topics such as a review of the National Patient Safety Goals and Joint Commission standards. I utilize an instructor-led class delivery system for topics that require more interaction and immediate feedback. For example, an intensive workshop on learning how to write for patients and families, incorporating plain language principles, is an instructor-led course that is four hours in length. Determining which delivery method is appropriate is done in collaboration with my education partner in the centralized education department within my organization.

Q **What are some of the key things you've learned about being a patient education manager? About patient education as a topic?**

A One of the things that I learned about being a patient education manager when I began my role in patient education was the vast amount of expectations and the diversity of skills needed to perform my job. As many patient education colleagues would tell you, it is often a lone ranger type of role, with you working solo to keep patient education alive. I choose the phrase "keep patient education alive" on purpose, because it is often just that—keeping patient education on the radar of senior leaders and staff members in order to ensure that it is delivered in an exceptional manner that ensures patient safety and satisfaction, and fighting for resources. Without those resources, patient education won't survive, at least in the sense of really making a difference. I've learned that in my role, I need to have both operational and strategic skills: I need to be able to effectively lead and facilitate meetings to accomplish end goals and strategize, as well as be able to carry out and implement that which I have set strategic goals for. I need to manage the day-to-day operations of patient education, such as chart audits, Joint Commission requirements, committee meetings, writing and editing patient education materials, and providing ongoing staff development opportunities such as classes and workshops. I also need to manage the strategic development of patient education by being a skilled communicator and negotiator, effectively in front of a group when discussing, vision and goal definition. I also need to be a highly skilled project manager for large projects that span several phases and several years, while at the same time implementing the projects I am managing. In essence, I've learned that you have to straddle the line and have one foot in operations, and one foot in strategy and do both very, very well virtually by yourself.

As far as patient education as a topic, I admit I started this role with very limited knowledge; I took what I knew about adult learning and transferred it to patient education, which was a mistake. I learned a lot on the job, reading often, and connecting with colleagues across the nation through the Health Care Education Association (HCEA). This is basically where all the patient education coordinators/managers "hang out," so to speak and bounce ideas off one another; it also helps tremendously to validate frustrations with the job, and where you're at. For example, I thought I worked slowly when it took me roughly 3 hours per page to edit/revise a patient education document. However I discovered this is an industry standard from talking with my fellow HCEA members.

Q How important is taking health literacy into account when educating a patient? Why?

A As mentioned above, health literacy, in my experience has truly defined patient education to a level that it wasn't previously. Assuming that all patient education is teaching adults in a hospital setting is an idea that, if left unchecked, can lead to unsafe health outcomes for patients. Health literacy opened many people's eyes to how patients learn and comprehend information, both in written and verbal formats. Health literacy also, in my opinion, forced both patients and providers to acknowledge just how critical effective patient education is to the health and well-being of patients. No longer is patient education just "a service" or another task that a nurse provides, but it's a critical necessity that helps to ensure the safety of patients, particularly after they leave our care. I know that when I was a staff nurse, I looked at patient education completely differently than I do now. It was definitely a task that needed to be accomplished, but I also assumed that everyone understood what I was saying; I assumed when I asked "Do you understand?" that patients answered openly and honestly. I didn't know what I didn't know. Health literacy is crucial to patient education and puts a different perspective on the task.

Q Do you think that the topic of patient education should be addressed more in medical schools?

A Without knowing the exact amount of hours that medical (and nursing) school curricula have dedicated toward the practice of patient education, I have to agree that more content about patient education should be incorporated, particularly components that address health literacy. I think that in discussing a crucial topic such as health literacy, the process of patient education naturally follows. Concepts about patient education (and its process) such as assessment, planning, implementing (teaching), and evaluating are covered when discussing health literacy and the importance of patients understanding health information.

Q What does The Joint Commission require as far as regulating patient education?

A The Joint Commission requires what I believe to be just the *basics* of patient education: to ensure that it is delivered, documented, and that key pieces of information are communicated. This is the minimum standard. The Joint Commission also requires that education is, in fact, individualized to each patient as evidenced by a learning assessment, evaluating barriers to learning and a patient's learning style preference. Again, in theory these aspects are all considered minimum standard. In practice, however, these elements are difficult to come by.

Q How do you ensure you stay in compliance with these regulations?

A Ensuring compliance is tricky and, dare I say, rarely are you ever at a point where patient education is in full compliance. In fact, when I first started in my role, chart audits were conducted that consistently revealed we were at 100% for patient education compliance. Upon further investigation, it turns out that 100% of the charts were showing documentation on the education flow sheet, but the Joint Commission required elements were not evident. So, first and foremost to ensuring that you remain in compliance is to conduct chart audits, being familiar with what The Joint Commission requires, so the audits are effective. The audits will reveal where the gaps or deficiencies exist. What specifically isn't being documented? The assessment? Patient goals? Depending upon what your audits consistently reveal, this will drive how you respond. Perhaps a staff in-service is needed. Perhaps it's a performance issue. Perhaps the practice needs to be underscored with an accompanying policy. Working closely with your system educator can help tailor your education needs and ensure you reach the goals you desire.

Q How does patient education relate to a hospital's bottom line?

A Patients who are not educated about their health and illness, and who do not understand what type of follow-up they need or how to take care of themselves, cost hospitals a lot of money. In fact, in terms of health literacy, it has been estimated that low health literacy costs the healthcare system $78 billion a year in unnecessary expenses. These expenses come in the form of repeat admissions to the hospital, such as the ICU for exacerbations of chronic diseases, including asthma and diabetes, or consistent use of the emergency department. Patients who do not understand how to take care of themselves will often be the "frequent fliers," utilizing health care services often for symptoms that could have been otherwise controlled at home or with the adequate self-care information.

Furthermore, since patient education is a requirement of The Joint Commission, failure to provide it could mean citations for the hospital, which means more staff time spent on remediation to resolve the discrepancy.

Also in the mix is the potential for litigation if patients are able to demonstrate that they did not receive the information they needed, which then resulted in harm/poor outcomes. According to the American Medical Association, there have been cases, particularly regarding informed consent, where patients have been successful in suing hospitals and receiving compensation for having informed consents delivered to them in a fashion that they did not understand.

Basically, patient education does affect a hospital's bottom line quite significantly. The challenge is demonstrating this direct relationship.

Q **What are some tips you can give fellow patient education managers for making a case for more resources and funding for patient education?**

A The most successful way to make a case, particularly for more resources/funding, is to recommend a proposal and use data to strengthen your case. For example, if you are in need of funding for translation services, demonstrating the percentage of Spanish-speaking patients would be helpful in demonstrating an increased need for translated material. In addition, other data to support your case, such as recent trends, requirements, etc., will help.

Making the case for more resources or funding means appealing to decision-makers in your hospital, such as senior leaders or other executives. Knowing how to get your point across and demonstrating "why" is an important skill to have when advocating for additional resources.

Q **Is it important for the person in the patient education role to have a title? Can a staff nurse take on this role?**

A A staff nurse can most certainly evolve into this role, but by no means can this role just be part of a staff nurse's regular patient care duties. Patient education needs to have the attention of the highest levels of the organization in order to succeed beyond the basics, and in order to do this, it's helpful to be a titled leader. In addition, it elevates the perceived importance of patient education within the hospital system and allows for it to be heard/discussed at important venues (such as key leadership meetings and strategy meetings).

Q What do you think may be in store for the future of patient education, as far as regulation and funding goes? Do you think it will always seen as merely a "nice to have" part of patient care?

A I think the awareness of health literacy has helped to elevate patient education overall, which in time will lead it to be recognized more as a "need to have" rather than a "nice to have." Organizations such as The Joint Commission, Leapfrog, and National Quality Forum all have issued white papers, guidelines, and other recommendations that take health literacy into account, which, from a patient education manager perspective, finally puts some "meat" behind what we have been advocating for a while. (Unfortunately, it takes these outside organizations paying attention to patient education to gain the attention of hospital leaders). I think with this new focus on health literacy, the practice of patient education naturally follows (or should follow) and, as such, facilities will look at their patient education practice and functions to be sure that the infrastructure is in place to support new measures or requirements handed down from these outside organizations. I also think that, with the current shift of healthcare, toward patients with higher acuity and earlier discharge, more reliance is placed upon patients and their families to provide care that was traditionally provided in the hospital setting or by licensed care providers. As such, more focus on home care (and, likely, patient education) and preparation for care at home will shift priorities and elevate patient education to a "need to have" level within healthcare.

Q Do you rely on peers/other patient education managers for guidance when facing challenges at your facility? If yes, why and how does their support help you?

A Absolutely. The patient education coordinators/managers within HCEA have been invaluable. As a new person in the field of patient education, joining this group and becoming involved would provide a large benefit. It lessens the feeling that you are all alone and offers a collaborative network through which you can bounce off ideas and get instant benchmarking data.

Q **How do you get staff members to be accountable for educating their patients?**

A A tough challenge, especially because staff members don't report to the patient education manager/coordinator, but the only way to make staff members accountable for educating patients is to have it clearly spelled out in job descriptions and measure it annually in performance reviews.

Q **How necessary is it to include a patient's family in the education process, and why?**

A Including the family is a critical step in the patient education process. Not only is including the family practicing patient-family centered care, but it's recognizing that in many cases, patients are often cared for upon discharge by family members, who rely upon the health information to properly care for their loved one.

FREE HEALTHCARE COMPLIANCE AND MANAGEMENT RESOURCES!

Need to control expenses yet stay current with critical issues?

Get timely help with FREE e-mail newsletters from HCPro, Inc., the leader in healthcare compliance education. Offering numerous free electronic publications covering a wide variety of essential topics, you'll find just the right e-newsletter to help you stay current, informed, and effective. All you have to do is sign up!

With your FREE subscriptions, you'll also receive the following:

- Timely information, to be read when convenient with your schedule
- Expert analysis you can count on
- Focused and relevant commentary
- Tips to make your daily tasks easier

And here's the best part—there's no further obligation—just a complimentary resource to help you get through your daily challenges.

It's easy. Visit *www.hcmarketplace.com/free/e-newsletters/* to register for as many free e-newsletters as you'd like, and let us do the rest.

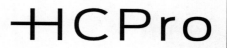 HCPro | Insight for healthcare compliance and management